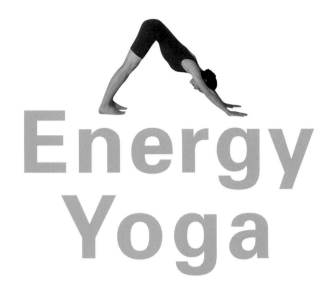

Energy Yoga

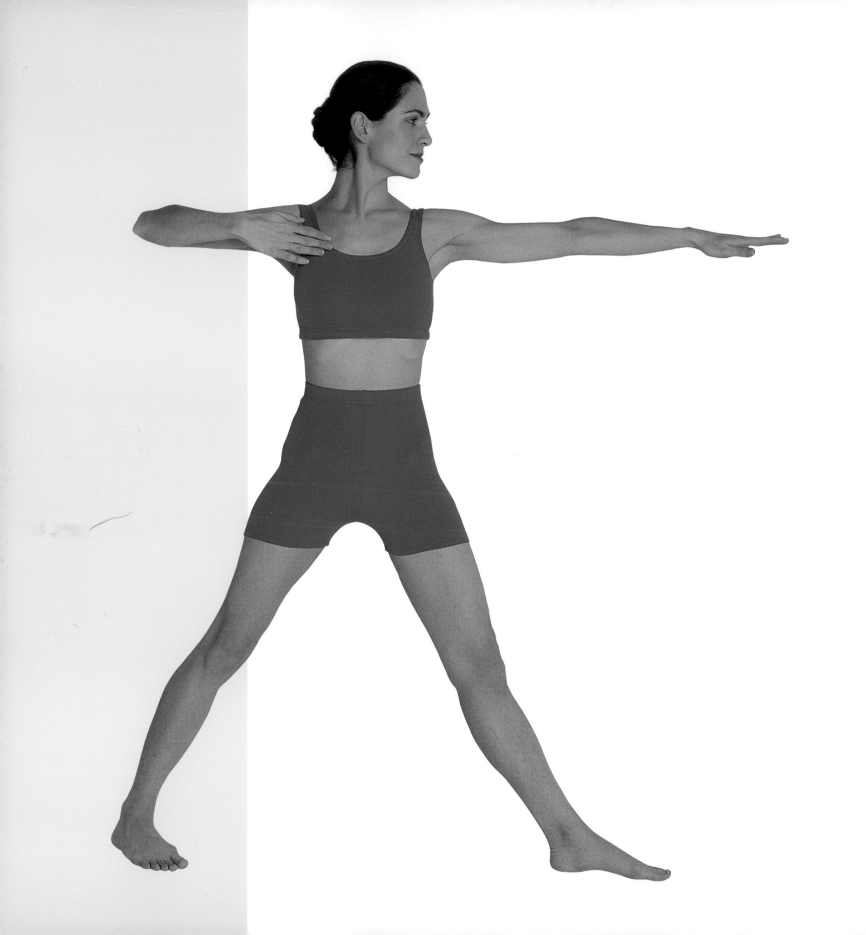

Energy Yoga

Emma Mitchell
Alistair Livingstone

DUNCAN BAIRD PUBLISHERS

LONDON

Energy Yoga

Published in 2003 by
Duncan Baird Publishers
Sixth Floor, Castle House
75-76 Wells Street
London W1T 3QH

Conceived, created, and designed by Duncan Baird Publishers Ltd

Material from this book was first published in the USA in 2000 by
Celestial Arts in two separate volumes from the *Naturally ...* series:
Energy Exercises and *Yoga for Energy*.

Managing editor: Judy Barratt
Editors: Ingrid Court-Jones, Kesta Desmond
Managing designers: Steve Painter, Manisha Patel
Designer: Rachel Goldsmith
Illustrator: Halli Verrinder
Commisioned photography: Matthew Ward

British Library Cataloguing-in-Publication Data:
Catalogue records for this book are available from the British Library

10 9 8 7 6 5 4 3 2 1

ISBN: 1-904292-80-1

Typeset in Rotis Sans Serif and Univers
Color reproduction by Colourscan, Singapore
Manufactured in China

Publisher's note
None of the information in *Energy Yoga* is meant as a substitute for
professional medical advice. If you are in any doubt as to the suitability of
any of the exercises or therapeutic methods given in this book, consult your
doctor. The publishers, the authors, and the photographers cannot accept
responsibility for any injuries or damage incurred as a result of following
the exercises in this book, or using any of the therapeutic methods
described or mentioned here.

"Everything rests in *prana* energy, as the spokes rest in the hub of a wheel." PRASHNA UPANISHAD

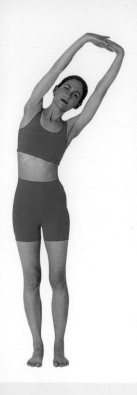

Contents

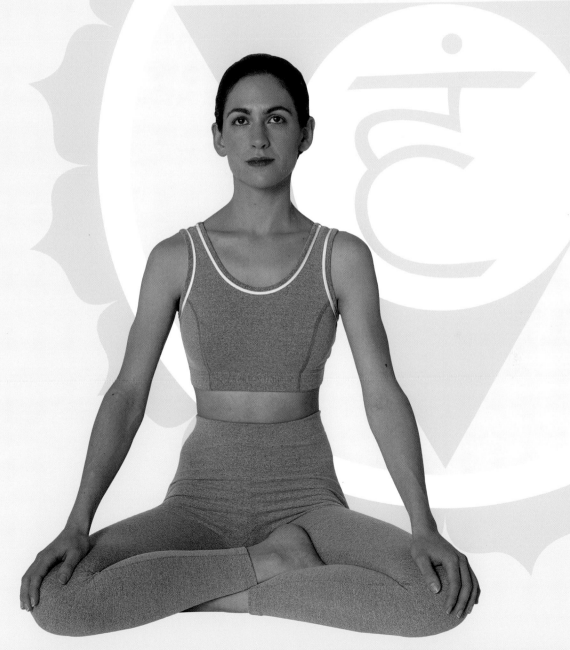

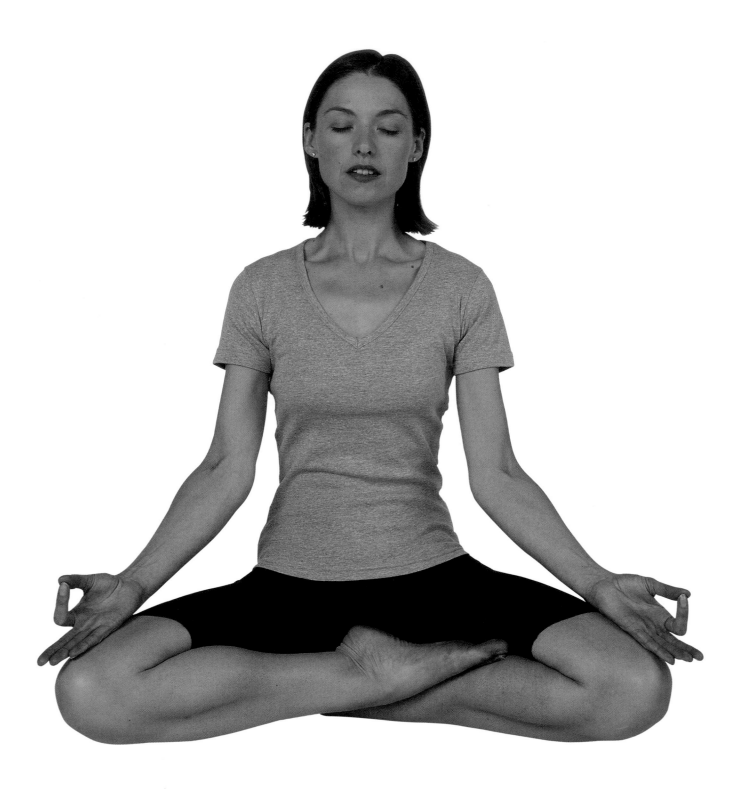

Introduction

Energy Yoga introduces disciplines such as t'ai chi, qigong and yoga, suggesting exercises, postures and movements to stimulate energy flow. It also features exercises based on the Western technique of kinesiology and on the therapeutic qualities of Egyptian dance. These disciplines acknowledge the existence of a vital energy that reaches beyond the physical to the essence of life and are increasingly recognized as ways to improve the appearance of the body, stay fit and prevent or treat long-term health problems.

You can practice all of the exercises found in *Energy Yoga* by yourself throughout the day, at home or at work, without the guidance of an instructor. The postures, breathing practices and relaxation techniques will help you to still your mind, revitalize your body, and restore your energy levels. Many exercises are modified for beginners, so that you can perform them easily and safely. By practicing the exercises in this book you can experience their energy-boosting benefits for yourself, and improve your health and happiness.

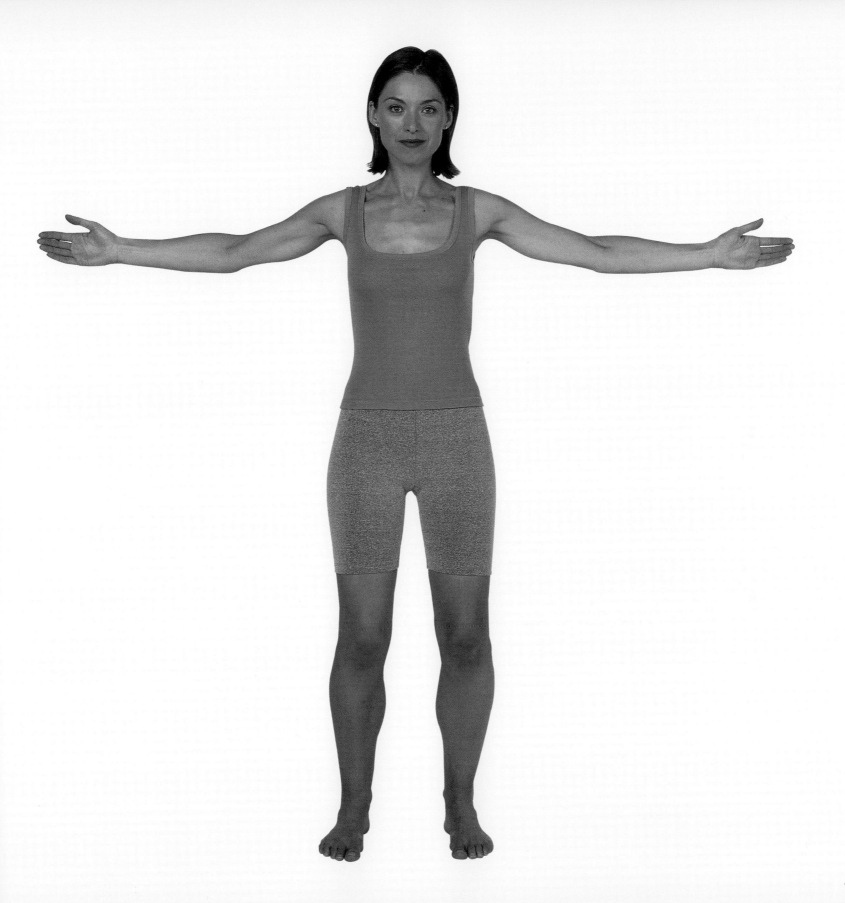

E NE
BALA

RGY
NCE

chapter one

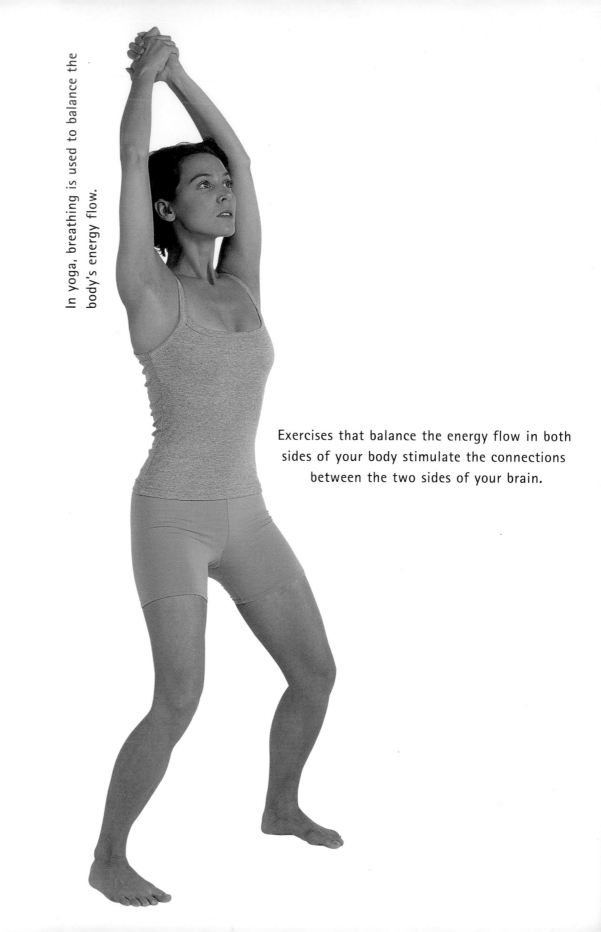

In yoga, breathing is used to balance the body's energy flow.

Exercises that balance the energy flow in both sides of your body stimulate the connections between the two sides of your brain.

Energy balance

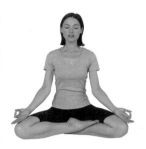

By stimulating the flow and restoring the natural balance of energy in our bodies, we can vastly improve the quality of our lives.

Energy flows through the body like a river and its tributaries, but often the stresses of Western living act like dams to cause flooding or drought, and disrupt the body's natural, harmonious state.

Imagine that you are able to summon up extra energy or switch off and relax at will. Imagine that your immune system reacts instantly to repel disease, and that you are nurtured with deep, nourishing sleep, and wake up feeling rejuvenated and eager to fulfill the potential of each day. When our body's energy flows freely and in balance, these benefits fall open to us.

Chinese wisdom

Balancing the flow of energy around the body has been the central aim of exercise disciplines throughout the Far East for centuries. In the Chinese traditions, energy flows along specific paths named meridians. There are said to be twelve meridians, each relating to a particular organ such as the stomach, the spleen, the kidneys and the liver. The body also has two reservoirs of energy known as vessels,

ENERGY BALANCE

16

which run up through the center of the torso and head (see p.21).

In China, energy is known as qi or chi (pronounced "chee") and is created by the tension between two opposing forces, "yin" and "yang". The male, yang energy is represented by the sun, and the female, yin energy is embodied in the earth.

There are three sources of qi. We receive congenital qi, which is stored in the kidneys, from both parents at conception. It is a barometer of our overall vitality, which can be depleted

by stress, lack of sleep and stimulants –
dark rings under the eyes are a sign of
low congenital qi. Nutritive qi enters
the body through the air we breathe
and the food we eat. Protective qi
surrounds our bodies. It prevents us
suffering from excess cold or heat, and
strengthens the immune system. To
enjoy good health we need constantly
to replenish our qi and encourage a
strong, balanced flow around the body,
by practicing energy exercises such as

t'ai chi and qigong and by breathing correctly, benefitting from the right amount of sleep, eating natural foods and drinking fresh water.

When we are affected by stress, emotional problems, shock or toxins, the meridians become blocked and this can cause imbalance in and impede the body's energy flow, in turn causing disease. This book includes some specific exercises for removing blockages (see pp.22-23).

Rivers of energy

the meridians

Each of our twelve meridians has two channels, one on each side of the body. The meridians form six pairs. One of each pair is a yin meridian, drawing up energy from the earth. This energy flows up the insides of the legs, up the body, and along the insides of the arms to the fingertips. The six yang meridians draw *qi* down from the sky, and the energy flows from the fingertips to the shoulders, head and body, and down the outsides of the legs.

Although we cannot see them, the meridians of the body can be measured electrically.
Tests have led practitioners to believe that they are located just under the skin.

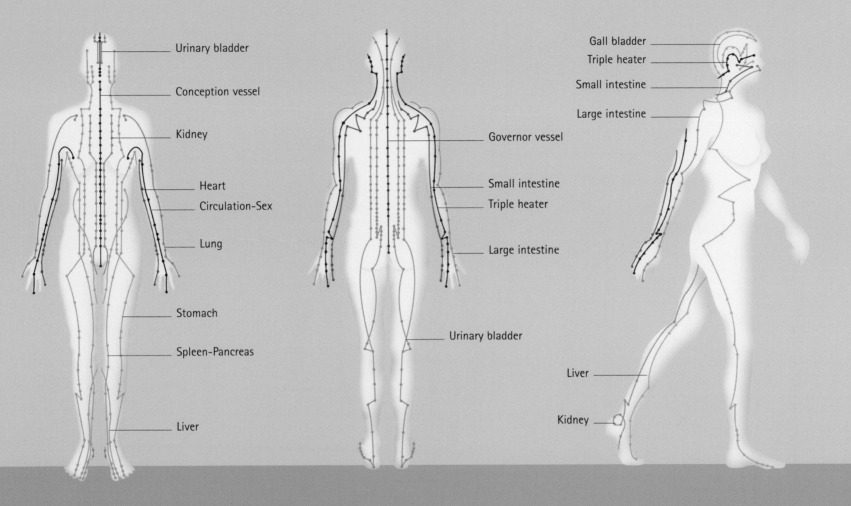

The meridians are all connected. The *qi* flows along them in a particular direction and around the body in a continuous cycle (see arrows in the key, right). The yin meridians are those of the lung, spleen-pancreas, heart, kidney, circulation-sex and liver; the corresponding yang meridians are those of the large intestine, stomach, small intestine, urinary bladder, triple heater and gall bladder.

Lung→ ● Large intestine→
Stomach→ Spleen–Pancreas→
Heart→ ● Small intestine→
Urinary bladder→ Kidney→
Circulation-Sex→ ● Triple heater→
Gall bladder→ Liver→

Governor vessel ● Conception vessel

Unblocking the meridians

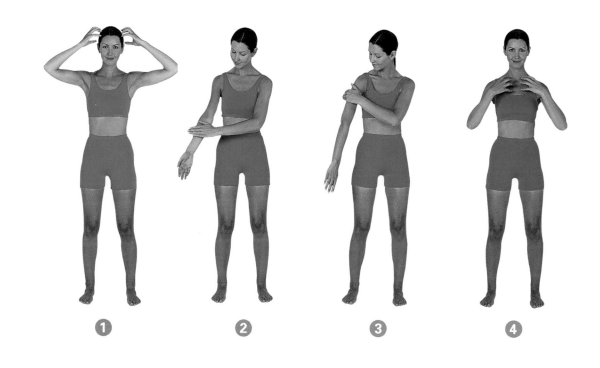

1 Tap all over your head with your fingertips, then stroke your hair. **2** Brush down the inside of each arm, from armpit to fingertips. **3** Brush up the outsides to the shoulders. **4** Tap your upper chest.

In this qigong exercise the hands sweep every meridian in the direction of the energy flow. In this way the movement of energy will break through any blockages, restoring balance and increasing vitality.

Launch into the day with this energy booster – it is especially good for banishing sluggishness in the morning.

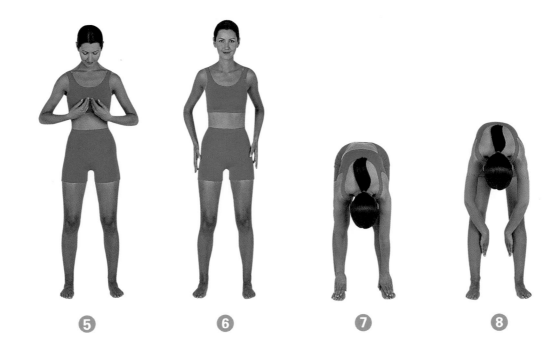

❺ Run your fingertips down your breastbone. ❻ Pat your hips and smooth down the outsides of your legs. ❼ Pass your hands over your feet. ❽ Continue up the insides of your legs. Repeat 10 times.

Qigong

The ancient Chinese tradition of qigong has a history stretching back more than 5,000 years. Today it is practiced by millions of Chinese to promote energy flow for health and spiritual wellbeing. The word qigong is made up of two Chinese words: qi, meaning energy or vitality, and gong, meaning practice. Together they mean "repeated energy work".

Stand, feet parallel, shoulders' width apart. Stretch your feet and splay out your toes. Your knees should be slightly bent and gently eased outward by your thighs. Gently draw up your abdominal muscles and allow your buttocks to sink toward the floor – from the waist down, your body should feel grounded. Lower your shoulders, drop your chin slightly to relax your neck, keeping your head erect as if it is being held from above. Let your arms hang down loosely, as if they were floating slightly outward. You should feel completely balanced and relaxed – if you feel any strain, try to ease it away as you breathe out.

Imagine that you are a tree. Visualize roots growing down from your feet, deep into the earth. You are tapping into the earth's goodness, which you draw up through your roots to nourish you. With each breath, you take in pure, positive energy to stimulate the flow of qi around your body and, as you exhale, you expel all the negative energy, toxins and anxieties into the earth, where they are absorbed and purified. You feel as if all your cares have melted away. Let your mind rest and feel at peace.

Qigong is said to be both subtle and internal: subtle because it is non-physical and intangible; internal because it focuses our energy inward.

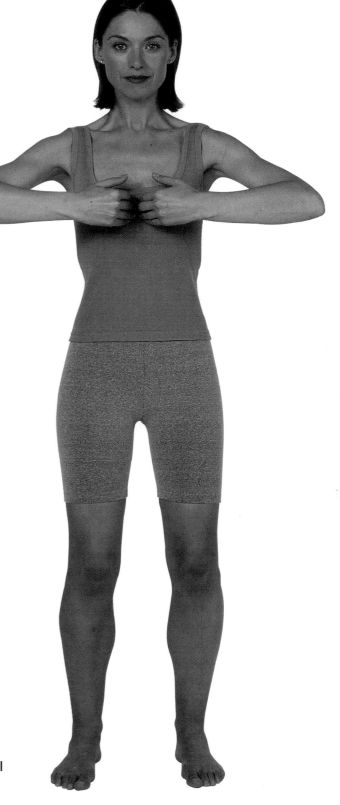

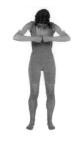

Achieving and maintaining balance

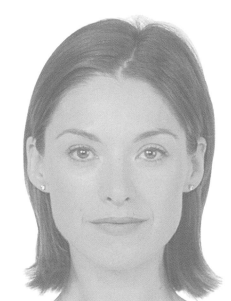

❶ Adopt the Qigong Basic Posture (see pp.25–26). Bring your elbows up and fingers in to the breastbone. **❷** Reach out your arms; keep your shoulders relaxed and imagine wrapping your arms around a huge ball of energy. **❸** Sweep your arms forward, squeezing the "ball"; bring your fingers back to your breastbone and drop your head forward. Repeat 15 times.

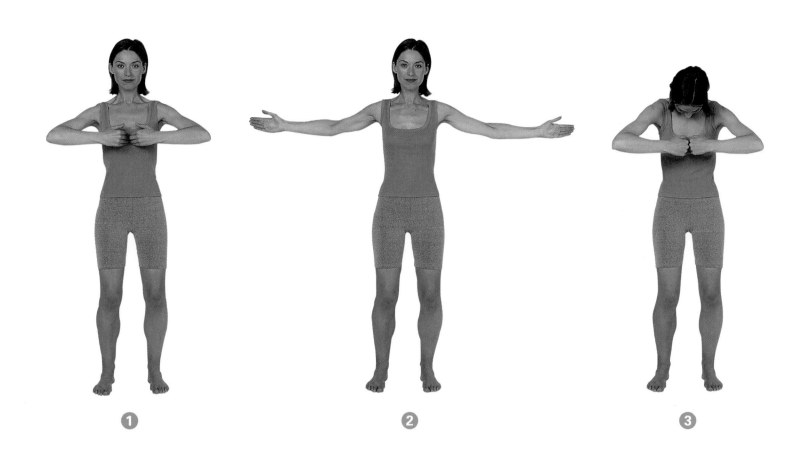

We often throw our bodies out of alignment by carrying a bag (or even our baby) with one arm, or standing with more weight on one leg, or always sleeping on one side. This exercise improves our bodies' symmetry, which opens up the central energy channel and balances energy flow around the whole body.

Ancient Chinese Daoists believed that a balanced flow of qi was the key to a long, healthy life.

Strengthening the energy flow

1 Stand, feet shoulders' width apart, knees slightly bent. Elbows out, bring your hands, palms inward, to your chest. **2** Stretch your arms out to the side. **3** Bring them up high above your head. **4** Cradle your skull in your hands. **5** Following the contors of your body, but without your palms actually touching your skin, sweep over your shoulders and down your chest to your lower ribs. **6** Sweep round to your back so that one hand is over each kidney. **7** Run your palms over your hips and down the outsides of your legs. Sweep round the front of your feet and up your inner calves and thighs, returning to the lower abdomen. Repeat 20 times.

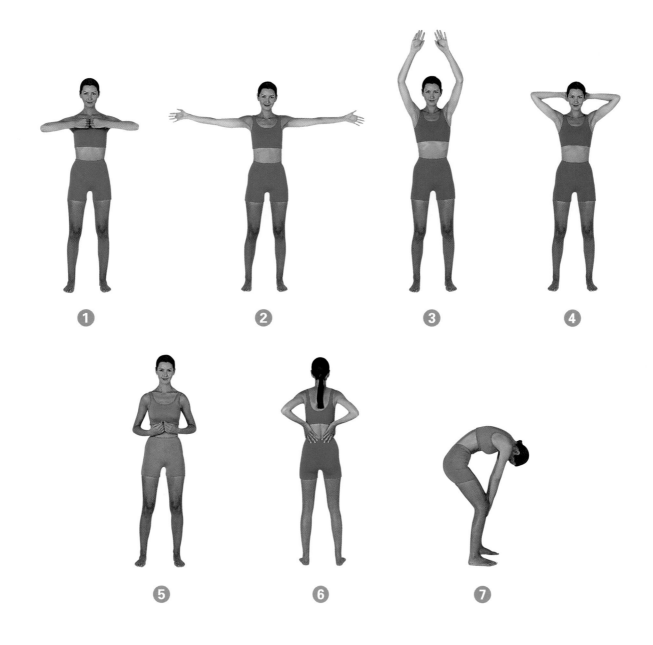

All meridian flow is stimulated by this qigong movement, but it particularly increases energy flow through the gall bladder (the outsides of the legs, hips and abdomen), the large intestine (the shoulders), and the liver, kidney and spleen-pancreas meridians, which run up the insides of the legs.

Sweep your body as the mood takes you: whether slow or quick, this exercise will keep your energy flowing strongly.

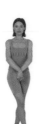

Visualizing energy

1 Standing with both feet planted firmly on the ground, cross your right leg over your left leg and your right arm over your left arm; now link your fingers together. **2** Keeping your fingers locked, twist your hands under and up, and at the same time press your tongue to the roof of your mouth. Breathe deeply, and visualize energy flowing around your body for one minute. **3** Keeping your tongue pressed into the roof of your mouth, uncross your arms and legs. Stand with your feet apart, bend your arms up and touch fingertips, then breathe deeply for one minute. Repeat the whole sequence, this time crossing your left leg over your right leg and your left arm over your right arm.

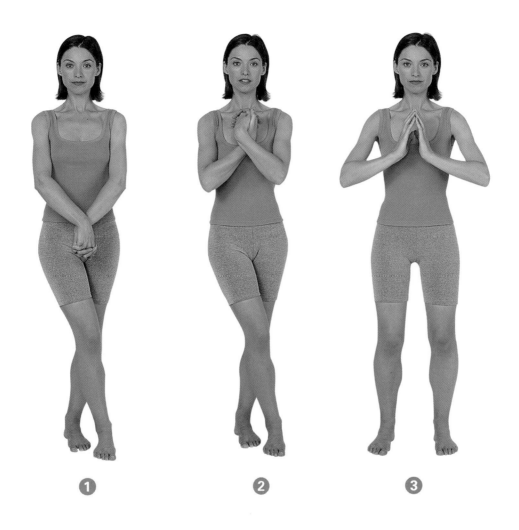

1   2   3

This kinesiology exercise, known as "Cook's Hook-up", is perfect to do first thing in the morning – it ensures that your energy flow is balanced from the very start of the day.

Go on! Kick-start your energy!

Our bodies have evolved so that they produce extra epinephrine when we are threatened. This makes our hearts pump more blood to our muscles to enable us to fight a predator or run away from danger. Today, we are more likely to face traffic jams than wild animals and, as aggression or escape are no longer appropriate responses, we tend to block the out-flow of excess energy, thus contributing to the build-up of stress. These exercises (pp.35–37) provide safe, alternative ways to release accumulated tension and re-establish your body's energy balance.

Fight or flight

the natural energy rush

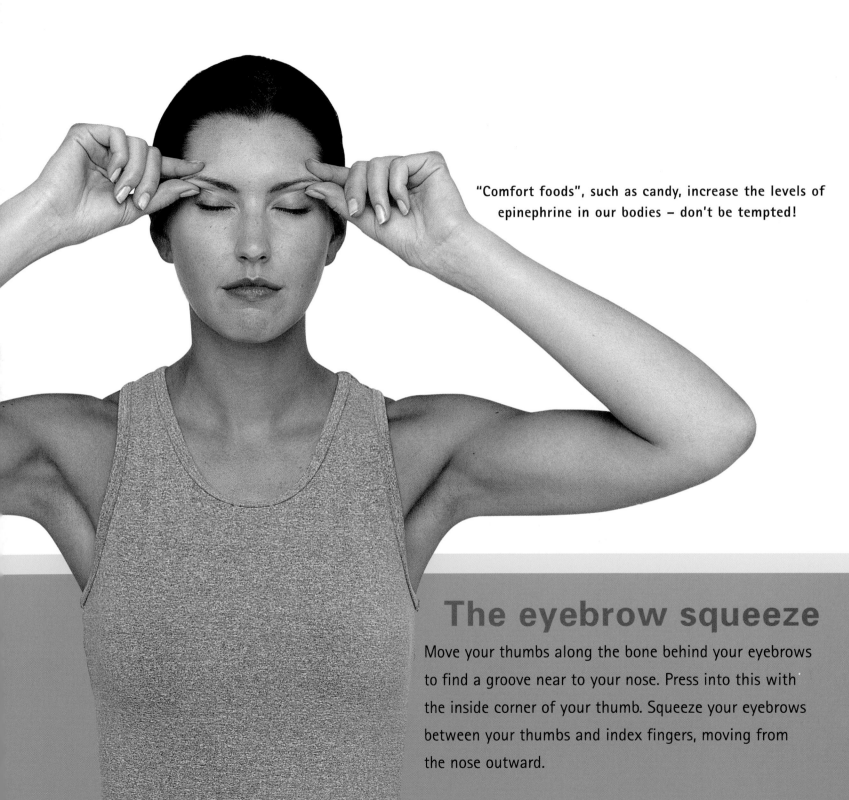

"Comfort foods", such as candy, increase the levels of epinephrine in our bodies – don't be tempted!

The eyebrow squeeze

Move your thumbs along the bone behind your eyebrows to find a groove near to your nose. Press into this with the inside corner of your thumb. Squeeze your eyebrows between your thumbs and index fingers, moving from the nose outward.

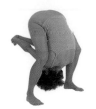 # The wood chopper

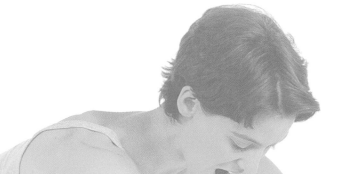

1 Stand, feet shoulders' width apart, knees bent. Clasp your hands together and lift your arms above your head, raising your chest and taking a deep breath. **2** Swing your arms down while exhaling and shouting "Ha!" as loudly as you can. **3** Keep the swing going until you have reached your arms as far through your legs as possible. **4** Swing your arms up again until they are high above your head. Repeat as many times as you feel are necessary to release any excess energy in your system.

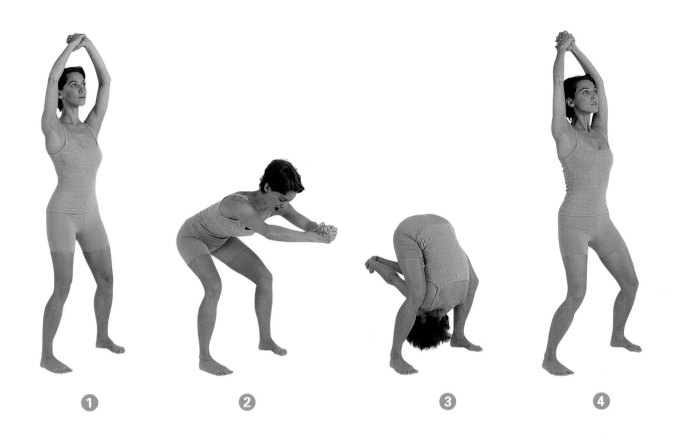

This polarity therapy exercise releases blocked energy from the solar plexus chakra (*manipura*), which if allowed to build up, can affect your judgment and cause indigestion.

Polarity therapy, developed by Dr. Randolph Stone (1890–1981), is a form of holistic healing, which treats the mind, body and spirit, and the energy system.

Paths to yoga

posture, breathing and meditation

Like traditional Chinese Medicine, the Indian practice of yoga teaches the importance of maintaining a free flow of energy around the body to ensure good health. Yogis advise living in harmony with nature, and balancing energy flow through posture and control of the breath. All yoga postures form a circuit of energy, and deep, quiet, regular breathing relaxes the body and helps to calm the mind. Yoga can include meditation – cleansing the mind of mental clutter, and stilling thought, often through focusing on a sound or a word (known as a mantra), or on a positive reflection.

There are four main paths to yoga: Karma yoga (Yoga of action), Bhakti yoga (yoga of devotion), Jnana yoga (yoga of knowledge) and Raja yoga (often called the "royal road"). Raja yoga is the mastery of mind and body

"Prior to everything, asana is spoken of as the first part of Hatha yoga."
Hatha Yoga Pradipika (1:17)

in order to release the higher nature. Hatha yoga is widely practiced in the West and is a sub-type of Raja yoga. The various postures and breathing techniques that form the basis of this modern practice are contained in the classic 8th- and 9th-century text, *Hatha Yoga Pradipika*. Hatha yoga includes posture (*asana*), breathing (*pranayama*), meditation (*dhyana*) and cleansing practices (*shatkarmas*). The *asanas* work on stretching and toning the muscles and skeletal

When the breath is irregular the mind is also unsteady, but when the breath is still, so is the mind. *Hatha Yoga Pradipika*

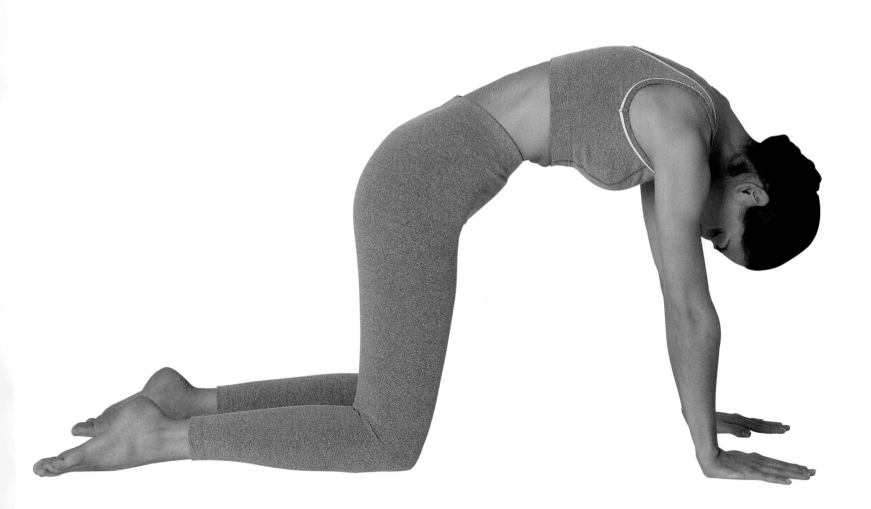

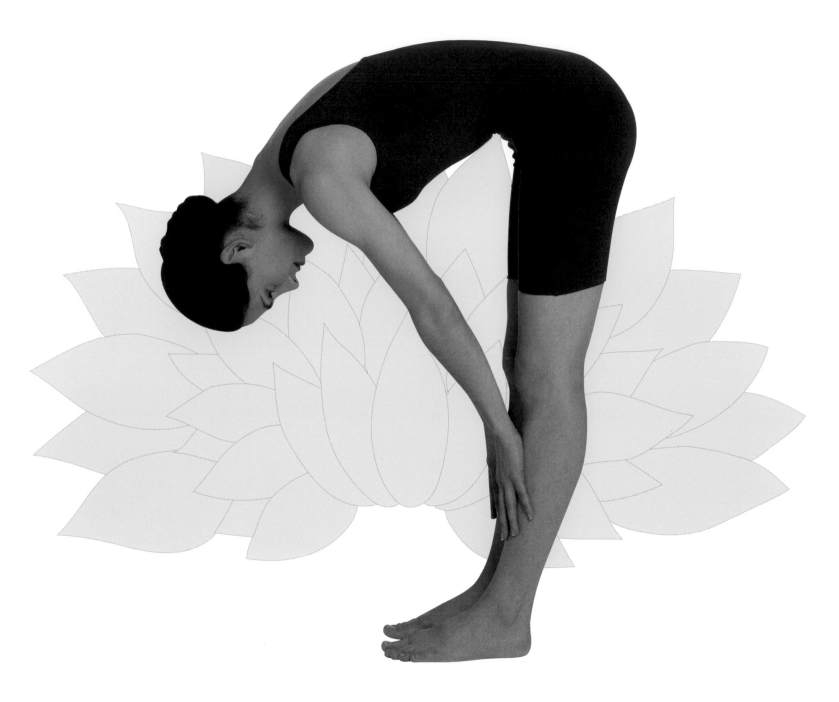

Having perfected the asanas, **one should practice** pranayama **according to the instructions of the teacher, with the senses under control, observing all along a nutritious and moderate diet.** *Hatha Yoga Pradipika*

framework of the body, as well as conditioning the organs and the nervous system. *Pranayama* practices calm the mind and revitalize the entire being. Relaxation and *dhyana* bring increased concentration and clarity. The cleansing practices of Hatha yoga, known as *shatkarmas* or *kriyas*, are very powerful and should be learnt only from a teacher.

Regularly practicing yoga helps to restore balance and harmony in the body and mind, removes toxins and releases vast resources of untapped energy.

Subtle anatomy

Western medicine tends to view the body as a collection of replaceable parts, many of which can be treated in isolation from one another. Other traditions view the body in a more holistic way, recognizing an essential inner energy, known as "life-force energy" or "vital force". In yoga teaching this energy is known as *prana*; when the balance of *prana* is disrupted, the result is illness. In yoga tradition the body has a system of chakras and *nadis* (channels) that generate and regulate *prana.* There are seven chakras on the midline of the body and many *nadis* through which *prana* flows.

"The removal of impurities allows the body to function more efficiently." *Yoga Sutras of Patanjali* (2:43)

Although chakras cannot be seen physically, they do have a relationship with the major physical organs in the body. They are positioned along the line of the spine. Many healers describe them as "spinning wheels of energy" and they are often represented by sound and color. The chakras are connected by three main *nadis*: *ida*, which passes by the left nostril; *pingala*, which passes by the right nostril; and *sushumna*, which runs up the middle of the spine. *Pranayama* and *asana* practice balances the flow of *prana*. Concentrating on certain chakras during *asana* practice can enhance the benefits of a posture.

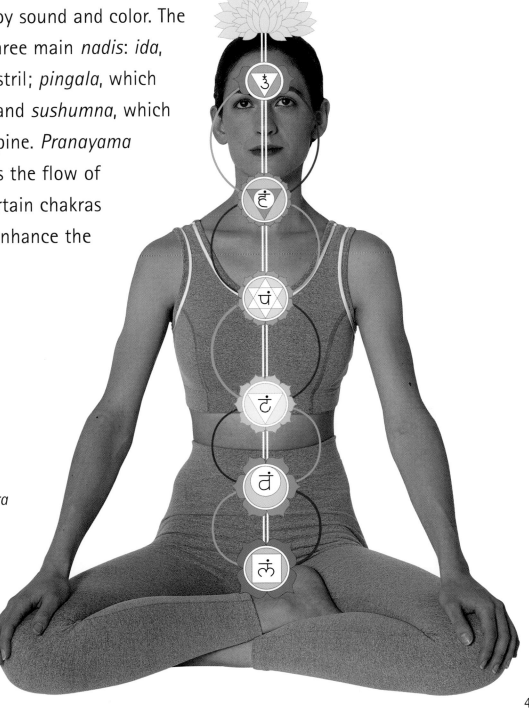

- Crown chakra – *sahasrara*
- Third-eye chakra – *ajna*
- Throat chakra – *vishuddhi*
- Heart chakra – *anahata*
- Solar-plexus chakra – *manipura*
- Sacral chakra – *swadhisthana*
- Base chakra – *muladhara*

- Left side – *ida*
- Right side – *pingala*
- Center – *sushumna*

45

Moving to stillness

Most of us live in a stressful environment. Some stress is useful – it drives us to meet our goals. Most of us, however, add unnecessarily to the stress in our lives; we often rush to and from work on busy transport systems, we carry too many bags, and we sit and stand in ways that make the body stiff and misaligned. Whether we are at work or at home, we spend much time sitting in front of a computer or television screen. All of these things sap our energy. Although it is impossible to banish stress entirely, we can learn ways to manage it. A main aim of yoga is to find a place of spiritual stillness from which to respond to the world: achieving stillness in postures and mastering your breath are vital steps toward this.

People often start to practice yoga because they wish to change something in their lives: to feel more healthy, be more positive, think more clearly, be calmer or have more energy. This impetus for change ultimately comes from a place deep within us that yearns to be quiet and content and free from judgment and blame. In Sanskrit this spiritual place is known as *purusa*.

Yoga is not about striving for the impossible – that is, attempting to achieve incredibly complex postures before you are ready. It is about working within your limits and developing a personal practice that brings you into contact with your internal energy flow and self-awareness. By learning to direct energy through the use of breath, the body, mind and emotions will come into harmony. This in turn leads you to a place of quiet and stillness, where decisions can be made with clarity and insight. Once you make contact with this place of stillness, you will notice that stressful parts of your life become more manageable. Make a commitment to live your life responsibly, fully experiencing each moment from a quiet place of understanding: this is yoga.

"The mind can reach the state of yoga through tireless endeavor and non-attachment." *Yoga Sutras of Patanjali* (1:12)

Relaxation posture

Shavasana is one of the most important *asanas* in yoga. You can use it to center yourself at the start of a yoga practice, and at the end as a final relaxation. You can also use it as a resting posture between more dynamic *asanas*. It is called the corpse pose because it requires you to lie perfectly still, and to slow your breath. This helps the mind to become quiet. Once you have mastered this posture, you can use it to relax at any time.

Lie down on your back, preferably on a blanket or a mat. You may need a folded blanket underneath your head for comfort. Visualize an imaginary line running from the top of your head to between your feet. Your body should be lying equally on either side of this line. Your hands should be about 6 in away from your body with your palms facing upward. Your feet should be 12–16 in apart. Lift your pelvis and lightly reposition it to let the spine lengthen. Allow each vertebra to relax and sink into the floor. Check that your head is straight and not to one side.

Now relax completely, knowing that your body and being are supported. Concentrate on the tip of your nose and focus on the breath as it enters and leaves the nostrils. Follow the breath up your nose then down into your throat and lungs. Imagine that you are floating above yourself, observing your body lying on the floor. Breathe "into" any points of tension, allowing them to dissolve. Finally, bring your awareness back to the tip of your nose. Think to yourself: "I know I am breathing in, I know I am breathing out."

If you have lower-back problems, you can make this pose more comfortable by putting a bolster or cushion under your knees.

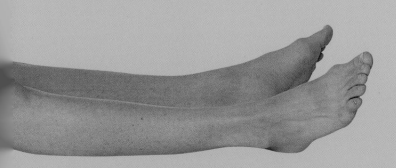

49

Simply sitting

Dandasana, the staff pose

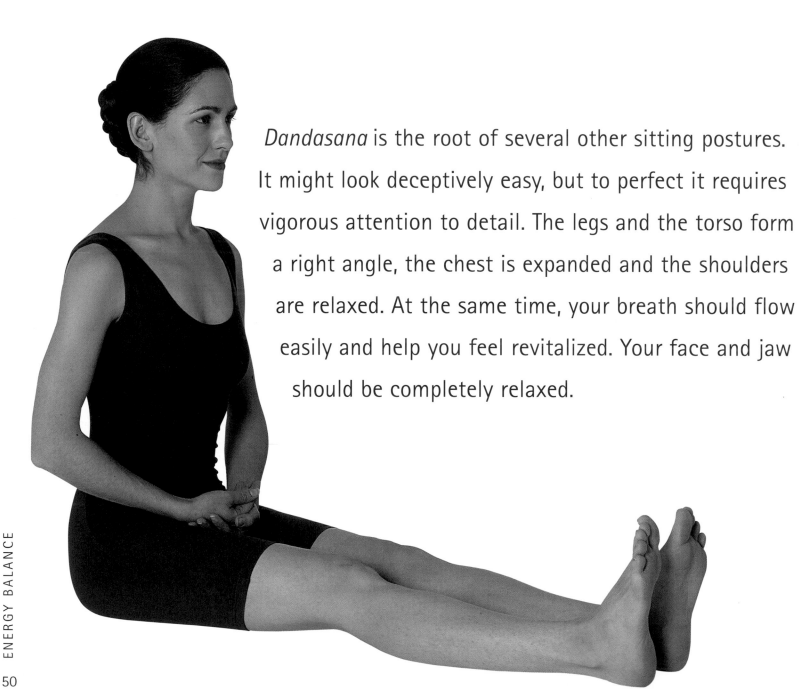

Dandasana is the root of several other sitting postures. It might look deceptively easy, but to perfect it requires vigorous attention to detail. The legs and the torso form a right angle, the chest is expanded and the shoulders are relaxed. At the same time, your breath should flow easily and help you feel revitalized. Your face and jaw should be completely relaxed.

Sit with your legs stretched out in front of you. Place your hands on the floor by your hips, either with your palms flat or on your fingertips. Supporting yourself on your hands, lift your hips off the floor and move the base of your spine back a little before lowering yourself again. You should now feel solidly rooted to the ground. Tighten your knees and stretch your heels away from you, with your ankles gently flexed and your toes pointing upward.

Press down on your fingertips and breathe in. Extend your spine upward, lengthen your lower back and imagine the top of your head is held on a fine thread. Open your chest area and lift your shoulders up and back. Breathe out. Let your eye muscles relax so that your focus is soft (or close your eyes). Now relax your jaw, cheeks, forehead and scalp. Release any remaining tension on each out-breath.

Raise your arms and make your hands into fists with your thumbs enclosed in your fingers. Breathe in. As you breathe out, flick your fingers outward, stretching them as far as you can. Then bring your fingers to the floor or fold your hands in your lap and return your awareness to your breathing.

Learning to sit without discomfort is fundamental to good yoga practice.

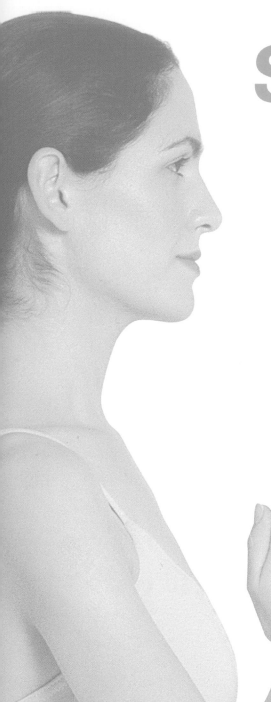

Standing tall

Tadasana, the mountain pose

We often overlook the energy-giving potential of everyday postures. Even an apparently simple standing position such as *tadasana* can be invigorating. The mountain pose helps to release tension that builds up imperceptibly in our bodies throughout the day. It may be considered one of the most fundamental *asanas* – the point of departure not just for the other standing postures, but for all yoga postures.

The idea of the mountain suggests stillness, strength and steadfastness – all crucial elements of yoga practice.

Stand with your feet close together, the inside edges parallel and nearly touching. If this is uncomfortable, move them apart slightly. Take your awareness down to the soles of your feet and feel the connection with the ground. Spread your toes. Shift your weight back a little and ensure that your heels are firmly on the floor. Imagine that you have strong roots that reach down from your feet into the earth, enabling you to draw energy up into your body, as with the Qigong Basic Posture (see pp.25–26). Visualize the energy flow as you tighten and relax each group of muscles and ligaments in turn: first the ankles, then the calves, knees (you may need to bend them slightly), thighs and hips.

Take a deep breath and, as you exhale, check that your lower limbs are relaxed. Tip your hips forward slightly, while gently pulling the abdominal muscles upward. Move your awareness to your diaphragm, chest and shoulders, and tense and relax each in turn. Take another deep breath in and raise your shoulders toward your ears. On your out-breath allow your shoulders to drop and relax. Imagine a fine thread gently pulling you by the top of the head toward the sky. Inhale, then say "ha" as you let the air out. Finally, bring your hands together in front of your chest in the prayer position, and breathe in and out, not controlling the breath but simply letting it flow.

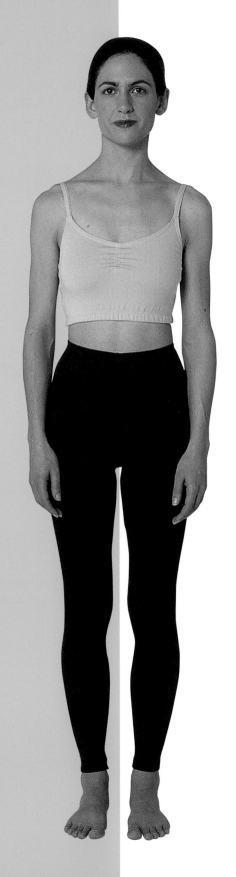

53

Yoga breathing

Pranayama

The key to releasing energy through yoga practice lies in the use of the breath. Because breathing is an automatic process, most of the time we are not aware of it and do not breathe to full capacity. *Pranayama* practice focuses awareness on the breath and the ability of pranic energy to revitalize the being. Most movements in *asana* practice are linked to in-breaths and out-breaths. Try to breathe through your nose, synchronizing each breath with the movement of your body.

Prana **means "vital force" or "life-force energy";** ayama **is defined as "expansion".**

Sit in a comfortable cross-legged position, press your palms on the floor and extend your spine upward, opening your chest. Place your palms on your knees.

Then place one hand on your abdomen at the level of the navel and breathe in slowly and deeply, allowing the abdomen to balloon outward. Breathe out slowly, using the abdominal muscles to contract the abdomen and expel all the remaining air. Repeat twice.

Now move both hands to the bottom of the ribcage so that the middle fingertips lie touching one another along the line of the lowest rib. Breathe in, expanding the ribcage as far as possible to the front, back and sides. Notice how far the fingers separate. (Check this again after a few months – you may find your lung capacity has increased.) Repeat twice.

Cross your arms and place your fingertips just below your collarbones. Breathe into the area at the top of the lungs, letting the breath come up as high as possible without straining. Let any tension drop away from your jaw or neck. Repeat twice. Now try to put the 3 actions together: breathe slowly and smoothly into the abdomen, ribcage and the top of the chest in one continuous inhalation. Then release the breath from the body. Repeat up to 5 times.

"Having gained control of the body through asana practice, pranayamas should be practiced." *Hatha Yoga Pradipika (2:1)*

Warming the body

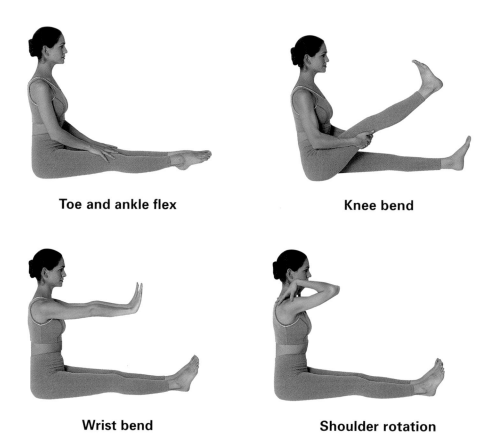

Toe and ankle flex

Knee bend

Wrist bend

Shoulder rotation

These warm-ups prepare the body for more dynamic postures by releasing energy blockages in joints and muscles. They can also help to alleviate rheumatism and arthritis, and are excellent for people who are advised not to practice more strenuous postures.

You can do these postures at home or at work, sitting on a chair or sitting on the floor – whichever is easier.

ENERGY BALANCE

56

Toe and ankle flex Breathe in and curl your toes back toward your body. Breathe out and curl them away. Repeat 5 times. Now do the same with your entire foot.

Knee bend Lift your right leg with both hands under the back of the knee. Breathe in and straighten your leg. Breathe out and bend your leg. Do not let your heel touch the floor. Repeat 5 times and then change legs.

Wrist bend Stretch your arms out in front. Breathe in and bend your hands back at the wrists. Breathe out and extend them forward and down. Repeat 5 times.

Shoulder rotation With your fingertips on the tops of your shoulders, rotate your elbows in a small circle. Make the circle bigger and include the shoulders in the movement. Breathe in as your elbows rise and out as they drop. Repeat 5 times then reverse direction.

FLEXII
AND M

BILITY
OTION

chapter two

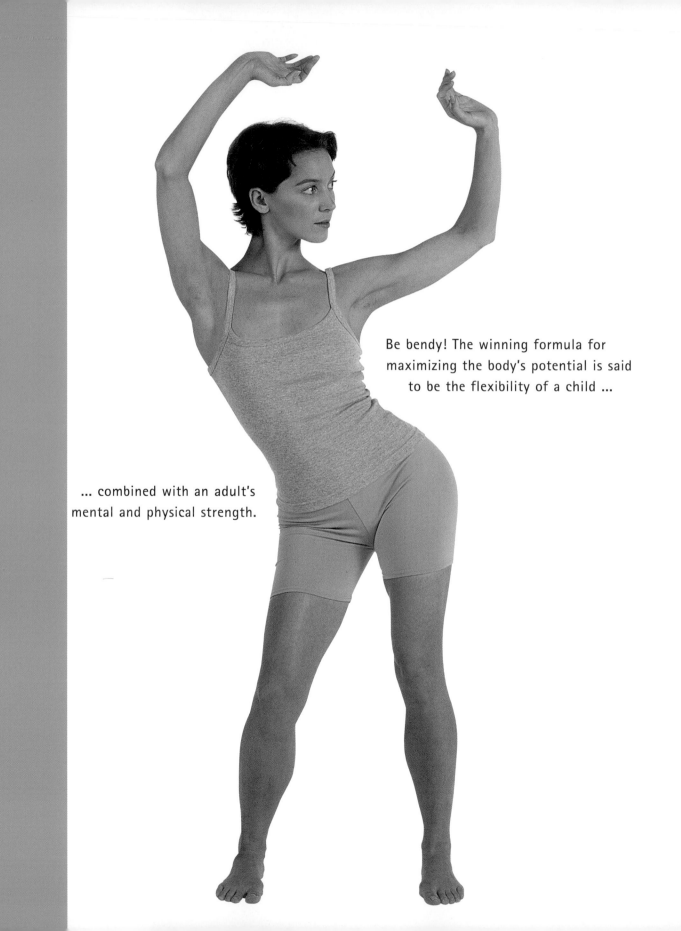

Be bendy! The winning formula for maximizing the body's potential is said to be the flexibility of a child ...

... combined with an adult's mental and physical strength.

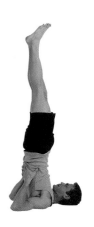

chapter two

Flexibility and motion

When we are conscious of our body's energies, we realize that during movement we are using energy to create more energy.

In the West the idea of exercise conjures up images of activities such as high-impact aerobics or jogging. Such strenuous workouts can impose stress on the body's joints and cardiovascular system. As a result, gentler types of exercise such as yoga, qigong and t'ai chi, which involve the use of static or slow-moving postures, and require mental as well as physical discipline, are gaining in popularity. Traditions such as these stimulate energy flow and make our movements more fluid as well as improving our overall fitness – without all the huffing, puffing, and exhaustion.

The waist swing

Much of the enjoyment in this t'ai chi exercise stems from
the graceful, rhythmical movement that increases energy flow.
It relaxes the upper body and calms the mind while toning the
abdominal muscles and massaging the internal organs.

Swing away stress! This exercise will loosen your shoulders and trim your waist.

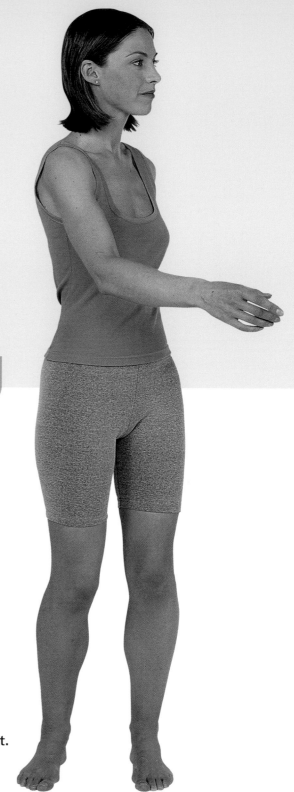

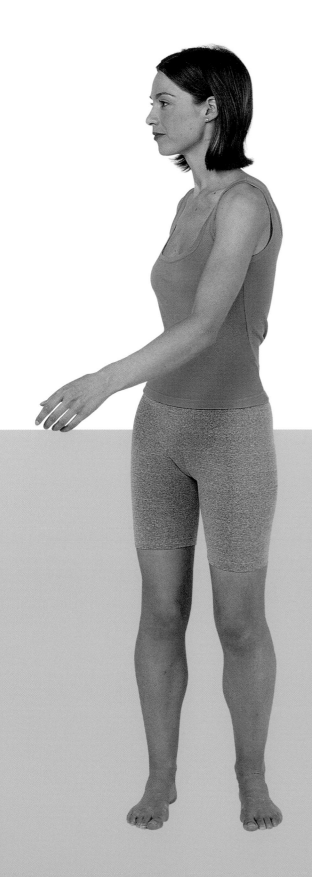

1 Stand, feet hips' width apart and flat on the ground, knees loose. Keeping the upper body relaxed and the arms floppy, thrust your right hipbone forward and your left hipbone back. **2** Return the swing by pushing your left hipbone forward and your right hipbone back. The twisting motion encourages the shoulders to follow and the arms to swing of their own accord. Concentrate on the hip motion and keep the upper body fluid. Continue until you feel warm and relaxed.

Pushing and pulling

1 Stand, feet shoulders' width apart. Inhale, raising your left elbow upward and parallel to the ground, the palm of your hand facing your chest. Raise your right forearm vertically, palm facing forward. Put your palms together. **2** Step forward with your left foot, pressing your right hand against the left, pushing the left hand forward beyond your foot as you exhale. **3** Use your left hand to pull the right one back. Inhale and bring your weight back onto your right foot. **4** Stand, feet parallel, shoulders' width apart. Elbows bent, open your arms with your palms facing forward and exhale. Repeat the whole sequence slowly, 5 times. Swap over to the other side.

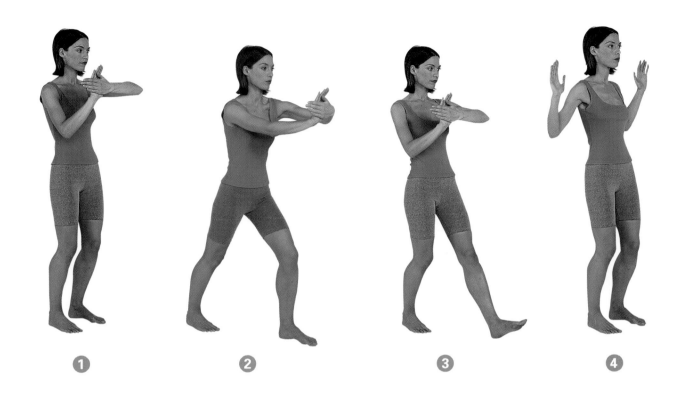

1 2 3 4

This t'ai chi exercise promotes the sensitive, flowing and reciprocal motion of energies
between the hands. It encourages awareness of the interplay between the opposing yet complementary forces
of yin and yang (for example, through pushing and pulling, controlling and yielding, giving and receiving) and
it helps to restore balance between the two forces.

**Practitioners of t'ai chi often benefit from a high level of flexibility well into old age – the gentle movements mean
that the exercises can be done by anyone, at any time of life.**

Movement to strengthen the legs

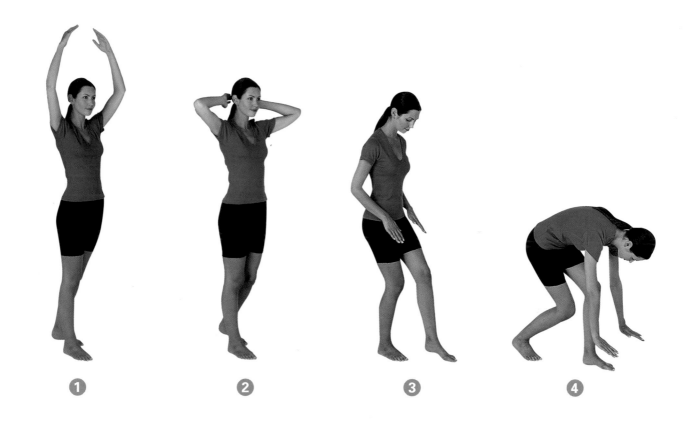

① ② ③ ④

This qigong walking exercise grounds the body's energy, promoting a good flow. It tones the muscles in the legs, shoulders and arms, and encourages increased flexibility and coordination.

According to the principles of qigong, each time we place a foot on the ground when we walk, we are reconnecting with the vital energies of the earth.

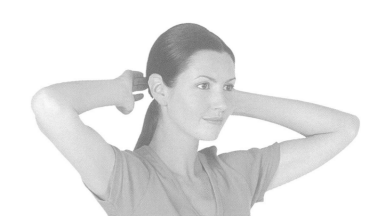

1 Step forward, put your weight on your right foot, your arms curved above your head. **2** As you begin to move your left foot forward, put your hands behind your head. **3** Sweep your hands over your shoulders and down to hip level as you move your left foot in front of your right and transfer weight onto it. **4** Lean forward at your waist, bend your knees and move your hands as far as you can toward the floor. Repeat 10 times, then swap legs.

Egyptian figures of eight

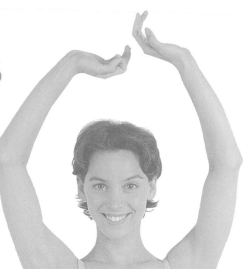

1 Stand, feet a little more than hips' width apart, firmly on the ground. **2** Keeping your knees slightly bent, move your right hip forward. **3** Push your right hip out to the side and then back, in a smooth circular motion. **4** Without hesitating, move your left hip forward. **5** Push your left hip out to the side and then back. Repeat, leading with alternate hips as if you are outlining a figure of eight. Maintain a rhythm, focusing on fluidly moving your hips while keeping your spine upright. Move your arms in the air to improve balance and add elegance.

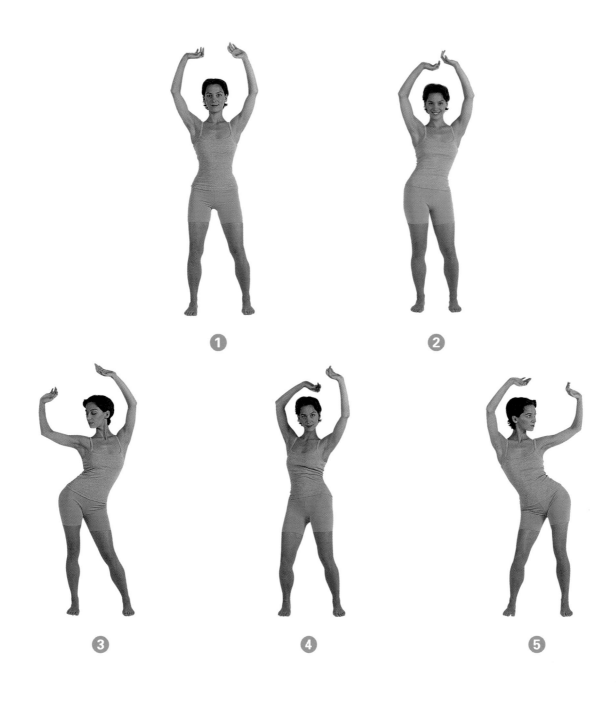

In Egyptian (or belly) dancing, the hips and abdomen move vigorously, leading the rest of the body, while the feet stay still – in this way the dancer maintains a connection with earth energies. Belly dancing tones the waist and hip areas and increases their flexibility. It also helps to heal pelvic, urinary, gynecological and digestive disorders.

"As long as there is life, there will be dance." (Margaret N. H. Doubler)

Egyptian hip drops

1 Stand with your feet hips' width apart, your right foot slightly forward. Keep your back and shoulders relaxed. Bend your left knee a little and raise your right heel, keeping the ball of your foot and your toes firmly on the ground. **2** Using your toes to push up, lift your right hip. **3** Bring the right hip forward and then lower it. Allow your arms, held above your head, to flow with the hip movement. **4** Sweep your right hip in a circle, from the front to the side and then back. Repeat Steps 2–4. Continue this sweeping motion for as long as you wish in a rhythmical and smooth movement. Repeat with your left hip for the same amount of time.

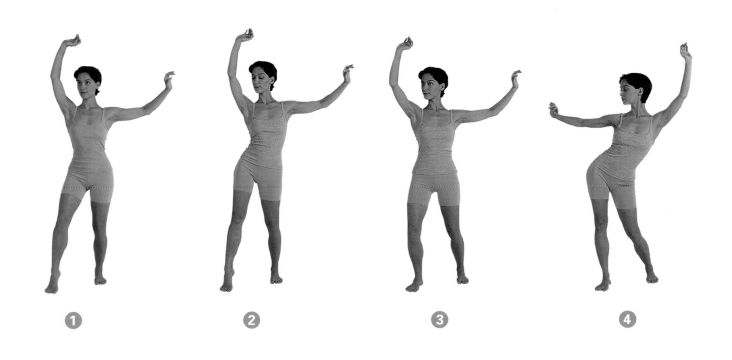

In this Egyptian dance exercise, energy flow is improved in the kidney, liver, urinary bladder, gall bladder, stomach and spleen-pancreas meridians, all of which pass through the pelvic area. Hip drops tone the abdominal, buttock and leg muscles, as well as greatly improving pelvic health and flexibility.

Dancing is healthy, therapeutic and enjoyable because it promotes flexibility in both
body and mind – to dance well we need let go and allow our energy to flow.

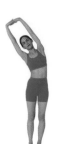

Arm stretches
tiryaka tadasana

1 Stand with your feet slightly apart, arms at your sides. **2** Stretch your arms out in front of you. Link your fingers, palms facing in. Breathe in. **3** Turn your palms out. Breathe out. **4** Breathe in and raise your arms slowly above your head. Stretch upward with your arms straight and your palms facing the ceiling. **5** Stretch to the right, extending the left side of your body. Breathe out. **6** Breathe in and return to center. **7** Stretch to the left, extending the right side of your body. Breathe out. Breathe in and return to center. **8** Breathe out and lower your arms to your sides. **9** Stand in the start position for a few moments then repeat the sequence twice more.

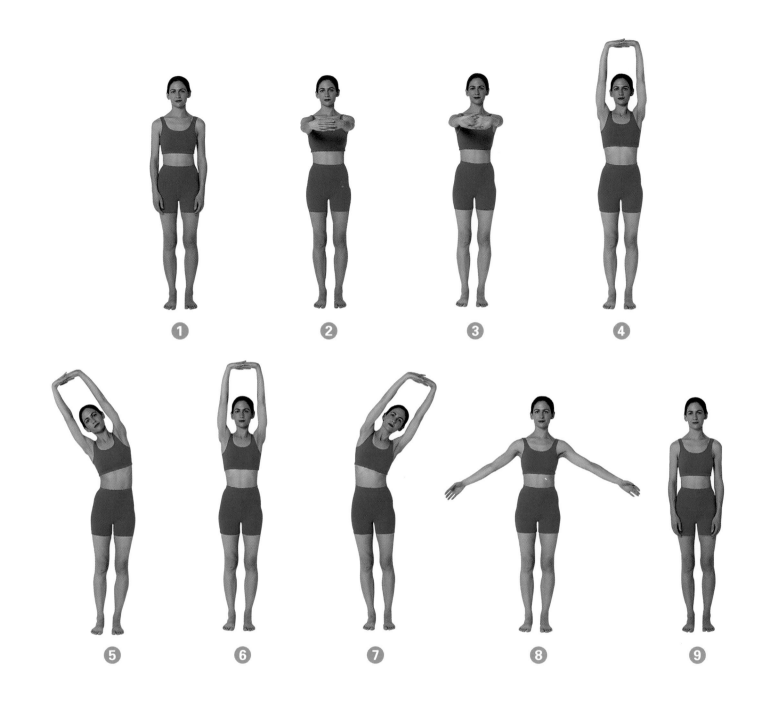

Stretching upward energizes the body, especially when accompanied by yogic breathing. Side stretches keep joints flexible and open the vertebrae laterally. In everyday life the spine is not usually extended in this way.

The movements of these arm stretches signify an ability to move the upper part of our body with the winds of change yet to keep our feet firmly planted on the ground.

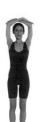

Forward bend
utthanasana

1 Stand with your feet slightly apart and your hands together in the prayer position. **2** Breathing in, raise both hands above your head, palms facing. Keep your arms straight and parallel, your fingers pointing up. **3** Breathing out, fold your arms above your head. Grip your elbows. Breathe in. **4** Breathing out, bend at your hips and knees as if going to sit down. **5** Bend forward and lower your palms to the floor. **6** Breathing in, let your fingers slide over your feet, ankles and the fronts of your legs. Straighten your knees and slowly stand up. **7** Breathing out, bring your hands back to the prayer position. Repeat the sequence, reversing the clasp of your elbows.

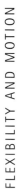

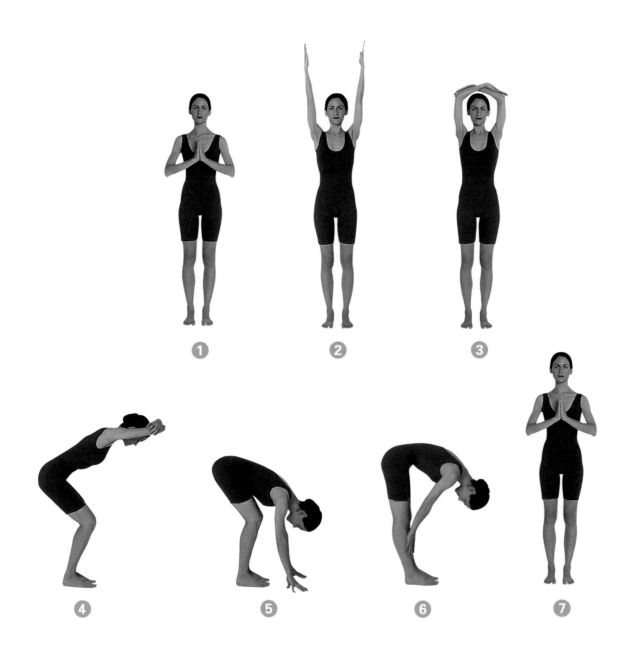

This *asana* sequence makes you feel refreshed and invigorated, and regular practice builds your energy levels so that you don't tire so easily. You should approach this sequence slowly. If you have any lower-back problems or suffer from high blood pressure, consult your doctor or a qualified yoga therapist first.

This sequence tones your back muscles and helps to make your spine more flexible.

The cat
marjari-asana

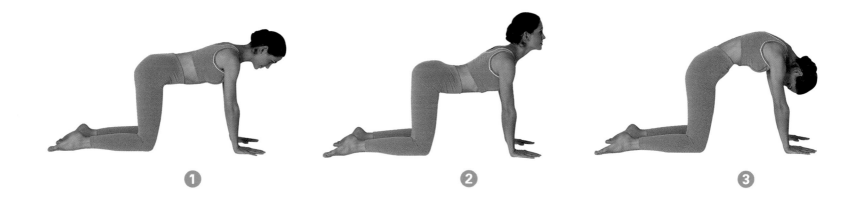

① ② ③

This posture frees the spine and neck, improves the circulation, and stimulates the digestive tract and spinal fluids. It is a useful posture for women who experience menstrual cramps. The Cat posture also teaches you to coordinate your breath with your movements.

When you practice this posture, focus on the eyebrow chakra (ajna) **as you breathe in and on the sacral chakra** (swadhistana) **as you breathe out.**

1 Start on your hands and knees. Your hands should be directly under your shoulders with your fingers spread out and your middle fingers pointing forward. Your knees should be directly under your hips, with your thighs at right angles to your calves. **2** As you breathe in, slowly roll your eyes upward and then raise your head, neck and shoulders to follow. Allow your spine to dip and your hips to tilt so that your tailbone points upward. **3** As you breathe out, pull your abdominal muscles up toward your spine and allow your hips to tilt forward and your head to come down so that your spine curves upward. Repeat this sequence up to 5 times.

Downward-facing dog
adho mukha shvanasana

1 Start on your hands and knees. Your palms should be shoulders' width apart and your fingers should be spread with your middle fingers pointing forward. Take a moment or two to breathe in and out, then curl your toes under your feet. **2** Breathing in, let your knees come off the floor – imagine that you are being pulled up into the air by the base of your spine. Keep your knees bent and allow your chest to come close to your thighs. **3** Breathing out, try to release your heels so that they sink to the floor. Straighten your knees and lift your hips. Relax your neck and shoulders. Keep breathing. Hold the posture for as long as you feel comfortable and steady.

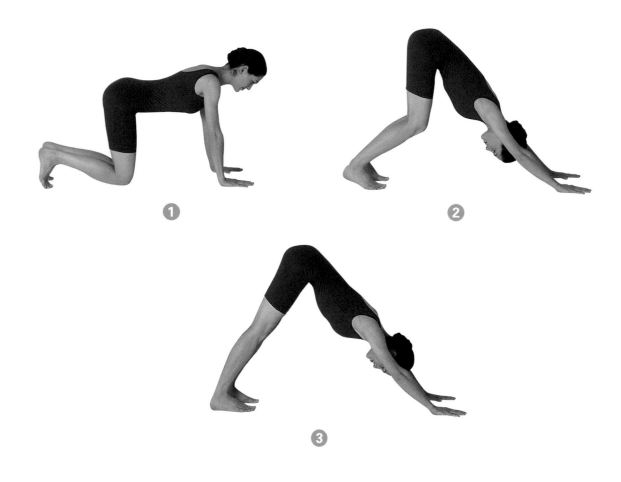

1

2

3

Downward-facing dog strengthens your arm and leg muscles, your spine and the long bones of your arms and legs. It also stimulates the circulation and nerves in the upper back and shoulders. When you practice this posture, focus your attention on the throat chakra (*vishuddhi*).

Yoga teacher Swami Ajnananda always used to remind his students that the Downward-facing dog is a posture in which they could meditate!

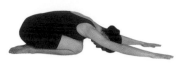 # Pose of the child
supta shashankasana

1 Start on your hands and knees. **2** Push back, sit on your heels and extend your arms. Gently rest your forehead on the floor. Feel the stretch and allow your spine to lengthen. Sink more deeply into the posture with each out-breath. **3** Make your hands into fists. Slide them back, resting one on top of the other under your forehead. **4** Sit back on your heels with your palms on your knees. **5** Breathing in, raise your arms in an arc in front of your body, above your head. Keep your palms facing in and your elbows straight. Breathe out and lower your arms. **6** Gently lower your forehead to the floor and extend your arms behind you, resting them by your sides.

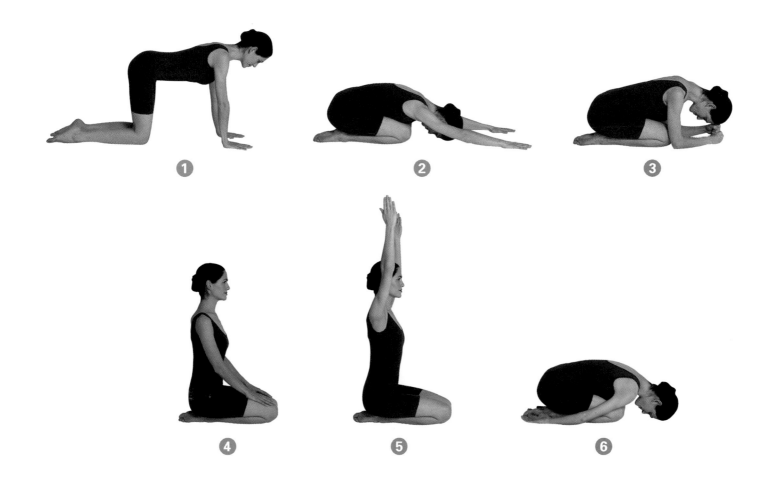

This series relaxes the spinal ligaments and stretches the back muscles. The final posture relieves compression on the intervertebral disks which become compacted when standing. It is a wonderfully relaxing posture.

If you find it difficult to sit back on your heels, try putting a cushion under your buttocks and sit on this. You can even try one under your feet as well.

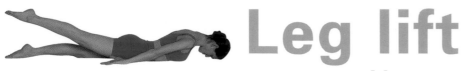

Leg lift
ardha shalabhasana

1 Lie face down and fold your arms in front of you, with one forearm on top of the other. Turn your head to one side and rest it on your arms. Focus on your breath – let it flow naturally. **2** Move your arms to your sides, palms facing upward. Your forehead should rest on the floor. **3** Breathe in and raise your left leg from the hip. Keep the knee straight. Breathe out and gently lower your leg. Repeat up to 5 times. **4** Repeat Step 3 with your right leg. **5** Press down with your arms and raise both legs together. Repeat up to 5 times. Return to Step 1 and rest with your head facing in the opposite direction.

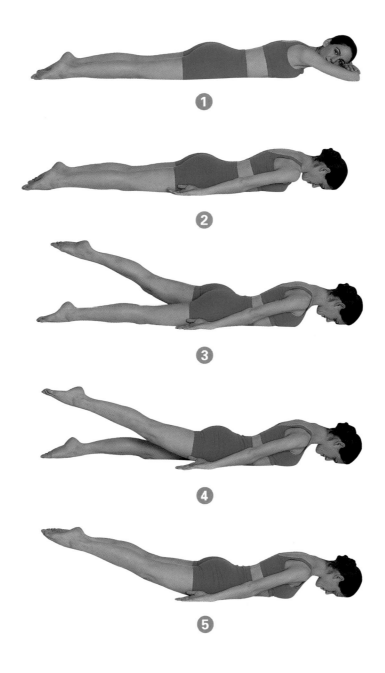

The Leg lift is helpful for beginners as it stimulates the nerves in the lower back and helps to strengthen the back muscles. Synchronizing breath and movement helps to develop concentration. When you practice the Leg lift, focus your attention on the sacral chakra (*swadhisthana*).

Don't attempt to lift both legs together until you are entirely comfortable raising the legs individually.

The cobra
bhujangasana

1 Lie flat on your stomach with your legs extended and your feet together. Fold your arms and rest your head on them. Relax your leg muscles. **2** Bring your hands underneath and slightly to the sides of your shoulders, with your fingers pointing forward. Keep your elbows close to the sides of your body and rest your forehead on the floor. Relax your whole body, particularly your lower back. **3** As you breathe in, slowly raise your head, neck and shoulders off the floor (your hips should remain firmly on the floor). Breathe out and slowly lower your body back to the starting position with your head facing in the other direction. Repeat this sequence up to 5 times.

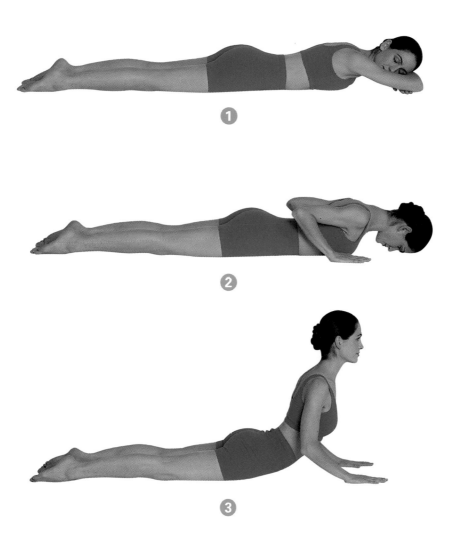

The Cobra strengthens the abdominal and back muscles and is beneficial for lower-back problems. It can also ease gynecological problems and, because it works on the abdominal organs, it aids digestion. It is a wonderful posture for activating energy from the base chakra (*muladhara*) to the third-eye chakra (*ajna*).

People with ulcers, hernias or intestinal problems should not practice this asana without expert guidance.

The thunderbolt
vajrasana

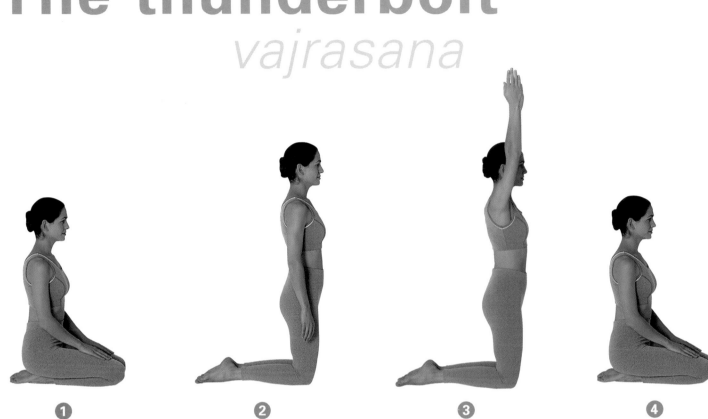

① ② ③ ④

Sitting back on your heels is a wonderful meditation posture for people who cannot sit cross-legged (even those with sciatica) and it activates life-force energy, or *prana*.

If you have varicose veins or poor circulation in the legs, place a cushion between your heels and buttocks to relieve pressure when you sit back on your heels. You may also find it helpful to put a cushion between the floor and your feet.

1 Sit back on your heels. Your insteps should be on the floor and your big toes should be touching, with the inside edges of your feet close together. Rest your hands palms down on your knees. Make sure that your spine is straight. **2** As you breathe in, come up from sitting into a kneeling position. Now breathe out. **3** As you breathe in, raise your arms in an arc in front of you, bringing your hands above your head, palms facing each other. Lower your arms in an arc as you breathe out. **4** Breathe in. Sit back on your heels as you breathe out. Repeat this sequence up to 5 times.

The butterfly
poorna titali

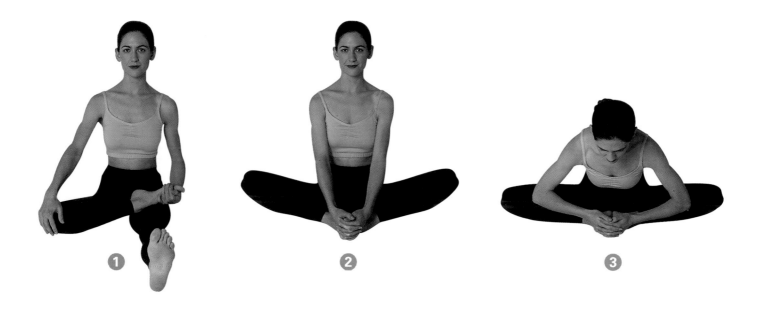

❶   **❷**   **❸**

This is a good preparation for the Lotus posture and for sitting in meditation. The Butterfly posture relieves inner-thigh tension and is helpful if you sit or stand for long periods.

It is said that the effect created by the movement of a butterfly's wings in one part of the world can trigger a tornado thousands of miles away. So be gentle in your practice!

1 Sit on the floor with your left leg extended. Rest your right foot on your left thigh, holding your toes with your left hand. Gently clasp your right knee with your right hand. Breathe in and out, raising and lowering your knee several times. Change legs and repeat. **2** Bend both knees and bring the soles of the feet together. Clasp your toes. Slide your heels toward your body. Straighten your spine and breathe in. Breathe out and lower your knees to the floor. Concentrate on counting your breaths and relaxing into the posture. **3** Bend your elbows and, working from the lower back, lower your body so that your chest comes toward the floor. Breathe in. Sit upright.

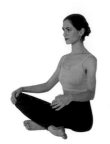

Easy spinal twist
sukhasana matsyendrasana

1 Sit with your legs crossed at the ankles, your back straight and your palms on your knees. **2** Breathing in deeply, raise your arms out to the sides. **3** Rest your right palm on your left knee. Breathe out. Turn your left palm to face backward. **4** Swing your left arm behind you and rest your palm or fingertips on the floor. Use this arm to help keep your spine straight and upright. **5** Breathing out, gradually turn your body to the left, feeling energy moving up the spine as you do so. Look over your left shoulder. Breathe in and out. Slowly release the posture as you breathe out. Return to Step 1 and repeat the sequence, twisting to the right.

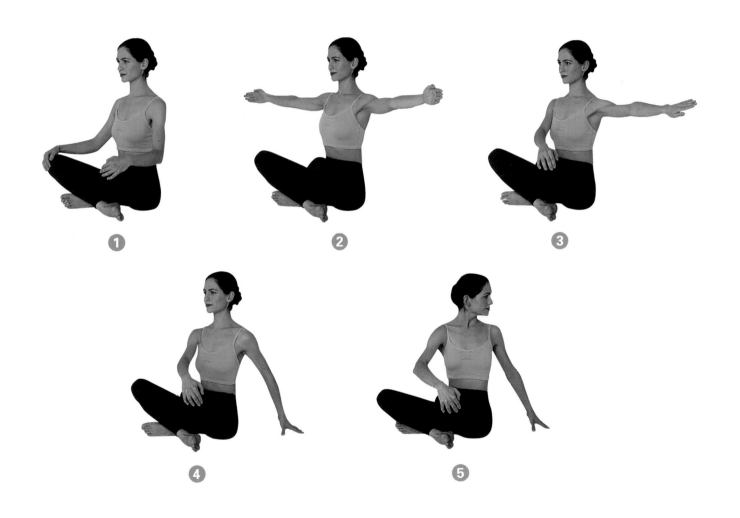

Twisting postures give the spine a wonderful workout, releasing enormous amounts of tension and flooding the spinal nerves with nutrients and energy. They open the heart chakra (*anahata*) and help to bring a greater volume of air into the lungs. They have a strong influence on the abdominal muscles as they stretch and compress them.

If you find it difficult to sit cross-legged on the floor, you can sit on a folded blanket or a firm cushion. Be careful not to over-extend yourself and twist more than your natural flexibility will permit.

The half-moon
ardha chandrasana

1 Stand with your feet slightly apart, breathe in and raise your arms above your head. Clasp your elbows. **2** Breathe out and bend forward at your waist, bending your knees if necessary. **3** Place your hands on the floor. Step your right foot back, keeping your heel off the floor. **4** Lower your right knee to the floor and straighten your toes. Breathe out. **5** Swing your arms forward and above your head. Keep your elbows straight and palms facing. Breathe in. Sink into your hips. Focus on your breathing. **6** Lower your palms to the floor and straighten both legs. Breathe out. **7** Swing your right foot forward and stand up. Repeat on the other side.

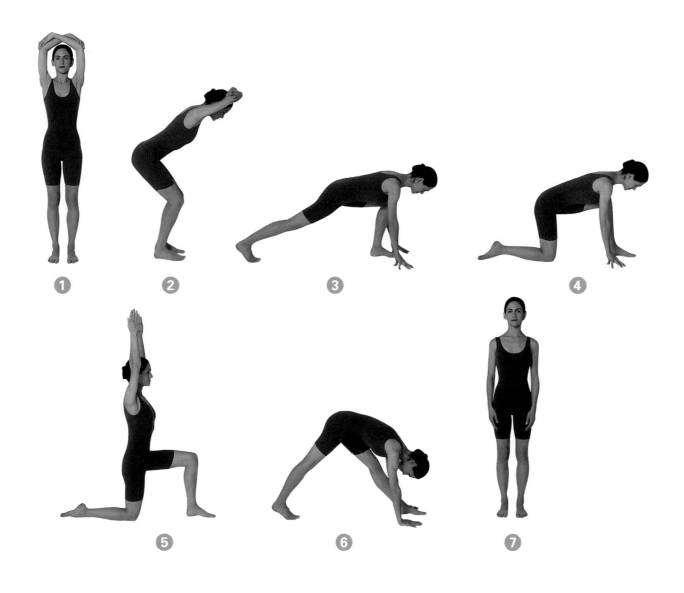

The Half-moon posture opens out the front of the chest and stretches the lungs. It strengthens the entire skeletal structure and, because it works strongly on the chest and neck, it frequently relieves respiratory ailments, including sore throats, coughs and colds. All in all it is a very invigorating posture!

When you practice this posture, focus on the sacral chakra (swadhisthana) **and on controlled movement and balance.**

The archer
akarana dhanurasana

1 Stand with your feet hips' width apart. **2** Step your left foot forward by a leg length and turn in your right foot so the instep aligns with your left heel. **3** Turn your hips and upper body to the right. Raise your arms sidewise to shoulder height. **4** Look along both arms – check that they are level with your shoulders. Extend your fingers. **5** Fold your right arm in toward your chest with your elbow at shoulder height, as if holding the string of a bow. Look along your left arm. Breathe in and out in the posture for as long as you can remain steady. Repeat on the other side.

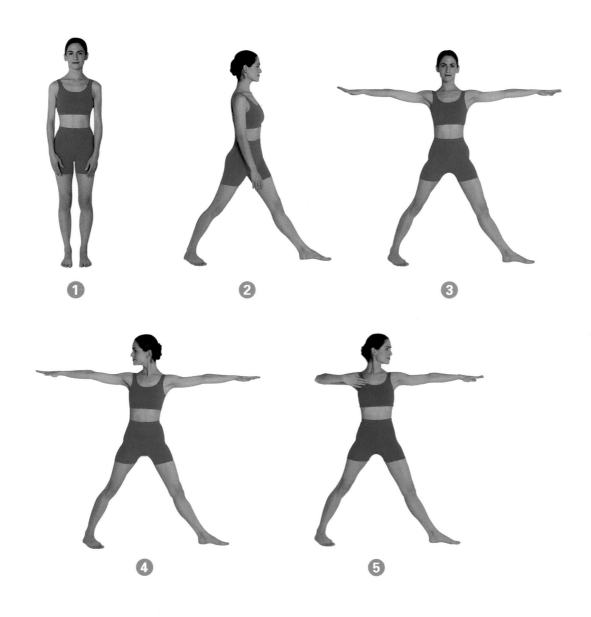

This posture works on the short, deep muscles in the neck and shoulders, and is excellent for releasing tension. To enhance tension release, try sliding the bent arm forward as you breathe out and bring it back as you breathe in.

Lord Krishna advised the warrior Arjuna to learn the wisdom of skill in action: "By this I mean perfect balance, unshakeable equanimity, poise and peace of mind." *Bhagavad Gita* (2:50)

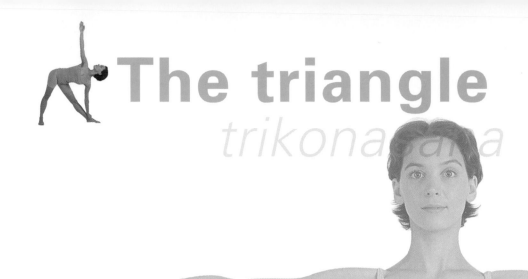

The triangle
trikonasana

❶ Stand with your feet wide apart. Breathe in. Raise and stretch your arms out to the side. **❷** Turn your left leg out 90 degrees and push your right heel slightly out to the right. Breathe out. **❸** Breathe in. Stretch your left hand down to hold your left ankle and your right hand straight up. **❹** Breathe out. Bring your right hand down past your right ear and stretch it out to the left. Breathe in. Stand up, arms outstretched. **❺** Lower your arms, and point your feet forward. Repeat on the other side.

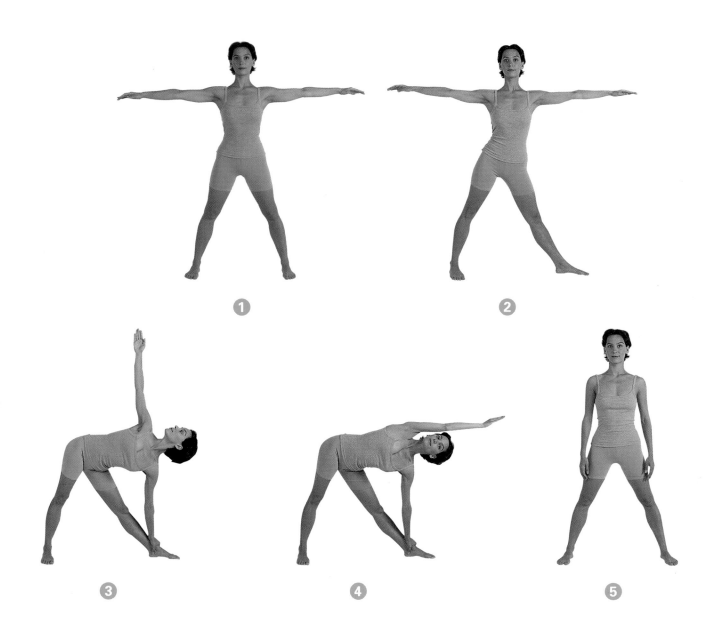

This yoga pose opens up the hip and shoulder girdles to allow the free movement of energy, and helps to trim the waist, making it more supple.

For maximum benefit take your time and do this exercise slowly – it creates a really satisfying stretch.

The bridge
kandharasana

1 Lie flat on your back with your arms near your sides and your palms facing down. Tilt your head slightly so that your chin moves toward your throat and the back of your neck lengthens. **2** Bend your knees and put the soles of your feet flat on the floor (first the left foot and then the right). Your feet and knees should be hips' width apart and your feet should be parallel. **3** Press down on your palms and, as you breathe in, raise your hips off the floor. Hold the posture. Breathe. Raise your hips a little more on each in-breath. **4** Breathe out and lower your hips. Stretch out your legs and then return to rest in the starting position. Repeat up to 5 times.

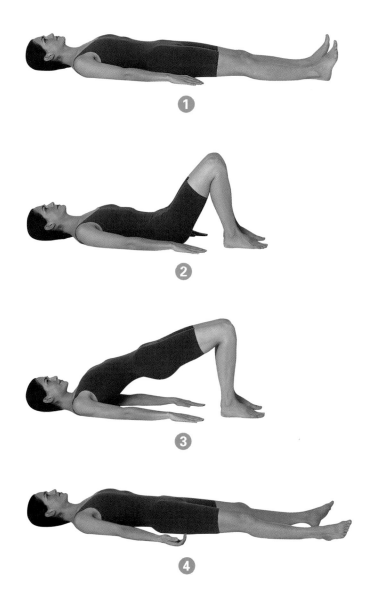

This posture massages the abdominal and female reproductive organs, improving digestion and easing menstrual problems. It can also help to realign the spine and relieve backache. People with ulcers or hernias and women in late pregnancy should avoid this posture or seek expert guidance.

When you practice this posture, focus on the heart chakra (anahata) **or the throat chakra** (vishuddhi).

The plank
setu asana

1 Sit on the floor with your legs extended, your spine straight and your hands at your sides just behind your hips. **2** Breathe in and lift your chest, gently arching your back. Breathing out, sit upright. **3** Take your hands a little further behind you so that your upper body is at about 45 degrees to the floor. Keep your arms straight. **4** Breathe in, roll your shoulders back and allow your chest to rise and your hips to lift off the floor. Gently point your toes, relax your neck and look up. Breathe. Try to raise your hips a little more on each in-breath. **5** Breathe out and lower your hips. **6** Gently lie down with your legs bent and your arms away from your sides. Relax.

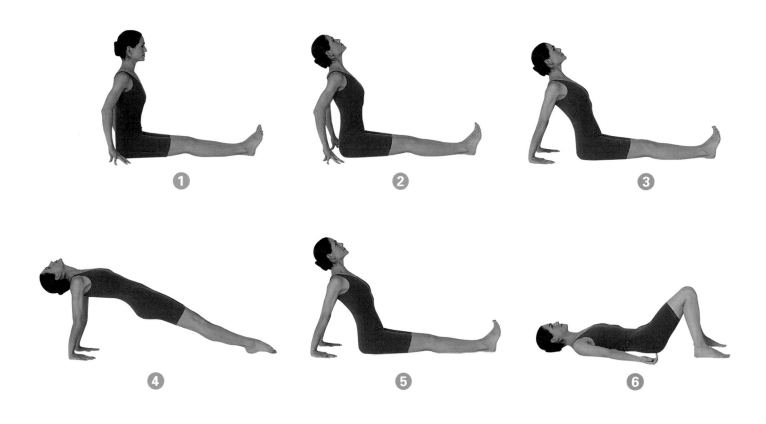

The Plank strengthens the arms, legs and the lumbar region of the spine. It is a good counterpose to forward-bending postures. You should avoid it, however, if you have high blood pressure, heart problems or a stomach ulcer. Focus on the solar-plexus chakra (*manipura*) during your practice.

When you can hold this posture comfortably, try lifting your pelvic area higher into the air. You can also try it with your hands facing backward and even lifting one arm or leg off the ground. Have fun!

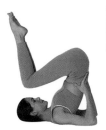

Half-shoulder stand
vipareeta karani

1 Lie on your back, arms at your sides, palms facing down. **2** Slide your feet toward your buttocks with your soles flat on the floor. **3** Push down with your hands and use your abdominal muscles to raise your knees. **4** Raise your legs and hips. Support your lower back with your hands. Your legs should be at a 45 degree angle to the floor, your feet relaxed and your elbows close together. Hold the posture and breathe. **5** Bring your knees to your chest, put your hands on the floor for support and slowly roll out of the pose, one vertebra at a time. **6** Lie down with your feet apart and your arms by your sides, palms facing up. Relax your body and breathe.

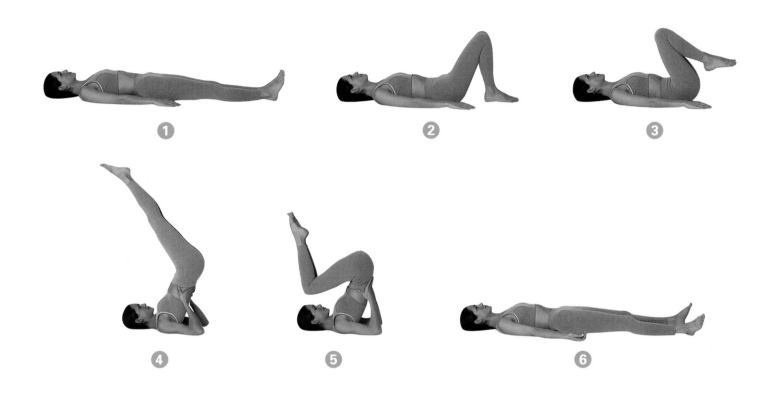

This posture stimulates the thyroid gland, relieves headaches and helps to calm mental and emotional disturbance. Do not practice it if you suffer from high blood pressure, weak blood vessels in the eyes or heart complaints. It should also be avoided during menstruation and the final stages of pregnancy.

"One achieves serenity by focusing on the inner light." *Yoga Sutras of Patanjali* (1:36)

The fish
matsyasana

1 Sit on the floor, legs extended, spine upright and hands behind your hips. **2** Breathing out, lower yourself to the floor using your forearms for support. **3** Slide your hands toward your feet. Raise your chest and rest the back of your head on the floor. Keep your chest raised as high as possible. Breathe in and out for as long as you are comfortable. **4** To release, slide your hands under your lower back, press down on your hands and elbows and lift your head. **5** Lie down. Release your hands, link your fingers and cradle your head in your hands. Pull your knees toward your chest. Cross your ankles and let your knees drop. Relax totally and focus on your breath.

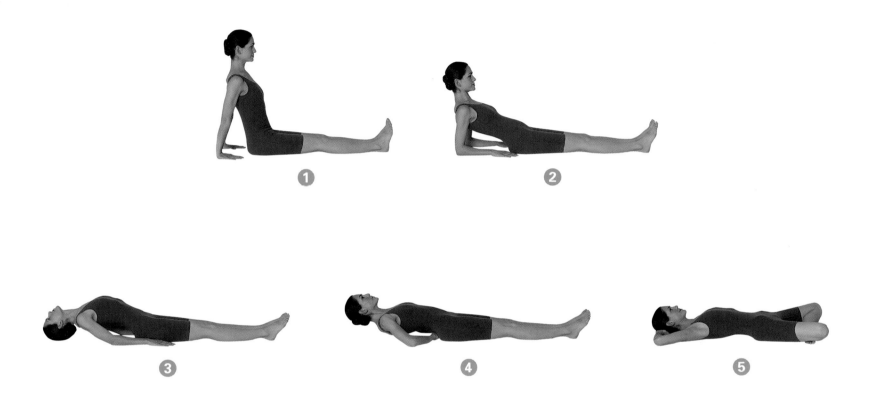

This posture opens up the chest and neck and is useful for abdominal and respiratory complaints, including colds and 'flu. It is also a very energizing posture. Take care getting in and out of this posture and avoid it altogether if you are pregnant, or suffer from heart disease or other serious health problems.

When you practice this posture, focus on the heart chakra (anahata) **in Step 3 and on the solar-plexus chakra** (manipura) **for the final relaxation.**

SUPER
YOU

RECHARGER DAY

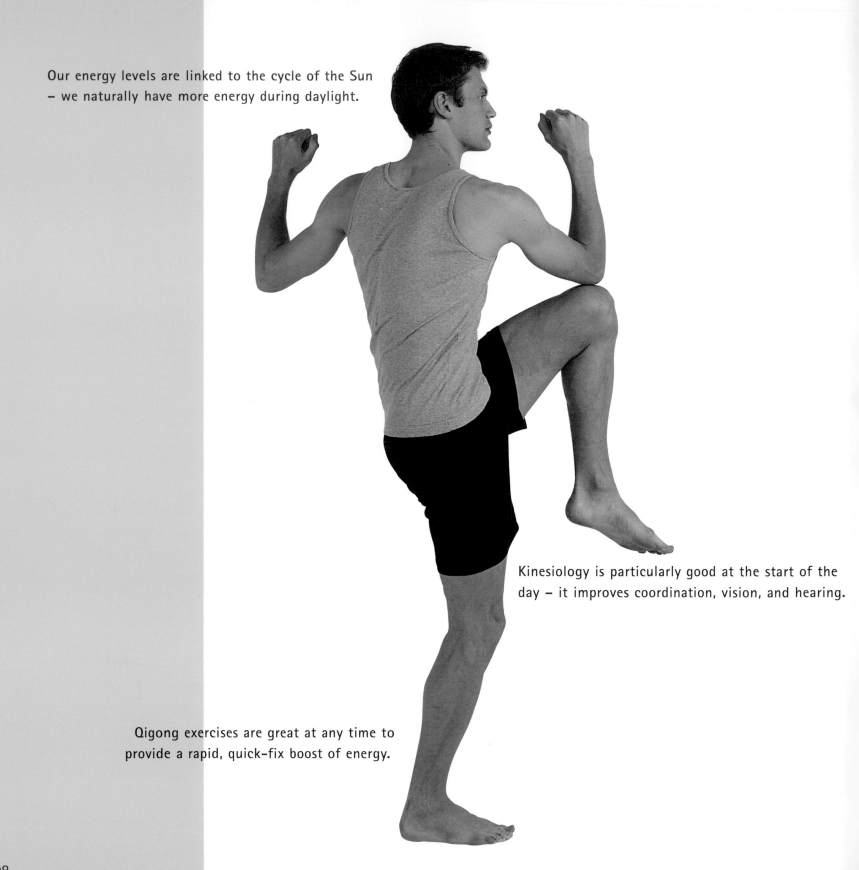

Our energy levels are linked to the cycle of the Sun – we naturally have more energy during daylight.

Kinesiology is particularly good at the start of the day – it improves coordination, vision, and hearing.

Qigong exercises are great at any time to provide a rapid, quick-fix boost of energy.

Supercharge your day

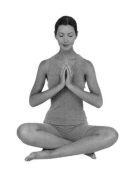

Understanding the ebb and flow of our energy levels through the day is important for living life to the full.

We all have different body clocks: some people feel sluggish and find it hard to function first thing in the morning; many have a dip in energy after lunch; and most of us feel drained at the end of a busy day. By learning to recognize and anticipate the fluctuations in our energy levels we can take steps to replenish our reserves to meet particular challenges at different times in our schedule. In this chapter there are exercises to improve our energy levels when we rise, after lunch and in the evening, as well as others that can quickly boost our energy flow whenever we need vitality most.

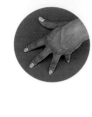 # The five-finger fix

1 Rest the tips of the thumb and four fingers of your left hand over your navel. Place the thumb and index finger of your right hand just below your collarbones. Wiggle all your fingers for 10 seconds to energize the meridians. **2** Keeping your left hand over your navel, place your right index finger on the middle of your top lip and your thumb on the middle of your lower lip, and rub these points for 10 seconds. **3** Place your right hand flat on the base of your spine and massage this spot for 10 seconds while still keeping your left hand over your navel. Repeat with your right hand over your navel and your left hand in the three positions.

ENERGIZE YOUR DAY

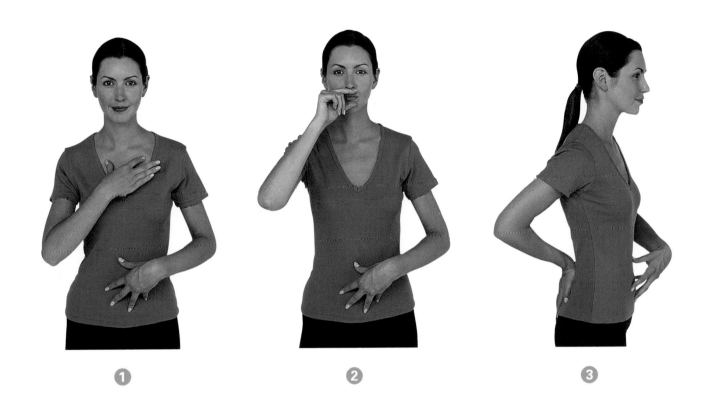

Massaging the two points below the collarbones helps to balance the energy flow in the kidney meridian. The fingers placed around the navel stimulate the flow of all the meridians in the navel area. The index finger and thumb placed on the lips connect the two energy reservoirs – the Governor and Conception vessels. The different actions of the two hands, and the points they massage, encourage the flow of electrical energy through the brain.

If you wake up feeling "out of sorts", kinesiology will point your energy back in the right direction.

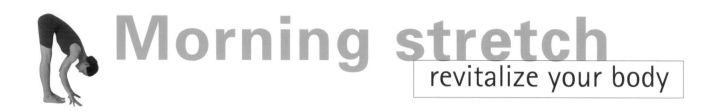

Morning stretch

revitalize your body

1 Stand up straight with your hands in the prayer position. **2** Breathing in, raise your arms in an arc above your head, fold your arms and clasp your elbows. Breathing out, bend forward at the hips. Extend your spine. **3** Lower your hands to the floor. **4** Step your feet back (right then left). Lift your hips up high and drop your heels to the floor. **5** Breathe out and bring your knees to the floor. Breathe in, raise your head, tilt your hips and let your spine hollow. **6** Breathe out, lift your abdomen, lower your head and look between your legs. Repeat Steps 5 and 6 twice. **7** Push back, sit on your heels and stretch from your fingertips to the base of your spine. **8** Sit upright. Put your palms on your knees. Focus on your breathing.

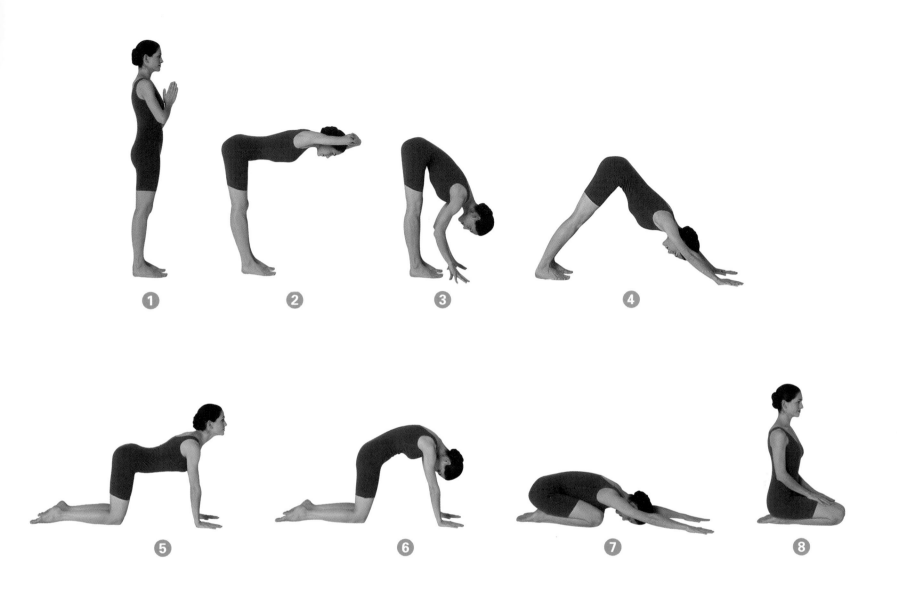

Give yourself at least 10 or 15 minutes for this sequence – it will invigorate you, balance your energy and prepare you for the day.

In the final stage of this sequence, close your eyes and make a resolution for the day. Open your eyes and smile.

The cross crawl

1 Lift one knee and swing the opposite arm so that the elbow touches the knee. **2** Lift the other knee and opposite arm in the same way. Looking at a plain wall, march like this 10 times, on the spot. Continue for another 10 marches, this time rolling your eyes widely in a clockwise movement. Repeat the sequence, this time rolling your eyes counter-clockwise. Now march another 10 times, moving your eyes in a large figure of eight. **3** Raise your right arm and right leg simultaneously 10 times, while following the above sequence of eye movements. Now raise your left arm and left leg, and march 10 times, repeating the eye movements once more. Finish by repeating Steps 1 and 2.

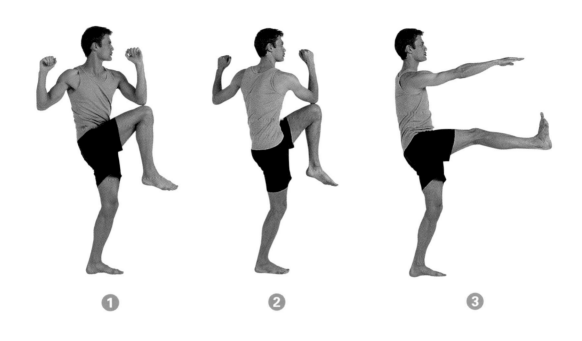

Kinesiology exercises are specifically designed to exercise the brain as well as the body. They improve the connections between the right and left hemispheres of the brain by coordinating movements between the two halves of the body. They are beneficial for everyone, but particularly for people with learning difficulties and dyslexia.

This exercise is based on, and named after, the crawling movements of babies.

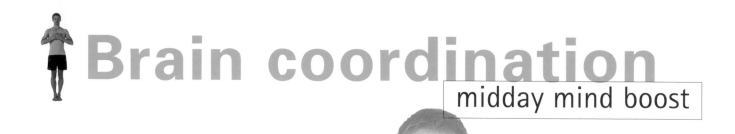

Brain coordination

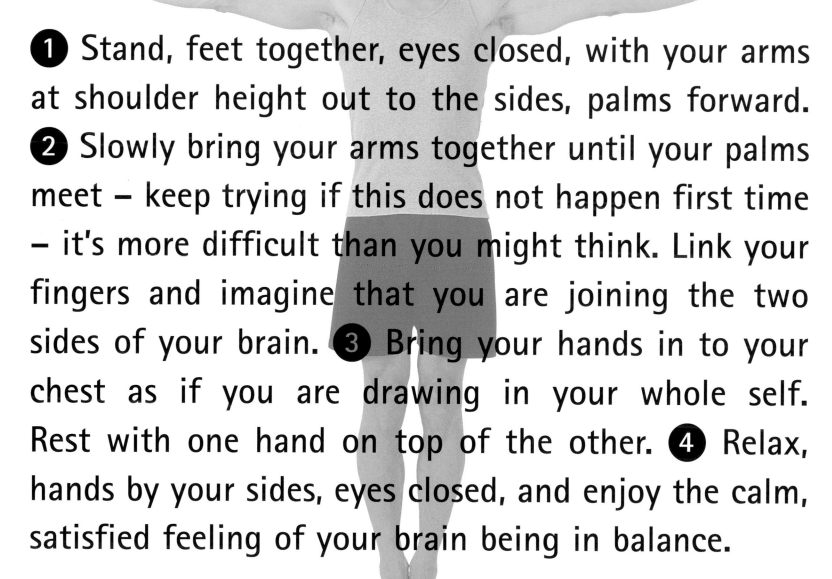

1 Stand, feet together, eyes closed, with your arms at shoulder height out to the sides, palms forward. **2** Slowly bring your arms together until your palms meet – keep trying if this does not happen first time – it's more difficult than you might think. Link your fingers and imagine that you are joining the two sides of your brain. **3** Bring your hands in to your chest as if you are drawing in your whole self. Rest with one hand on top of the other. **4** Relax, hands by your sides, eyes closed, and enjoy the calm, satisfied feeling of your brain being in balance.

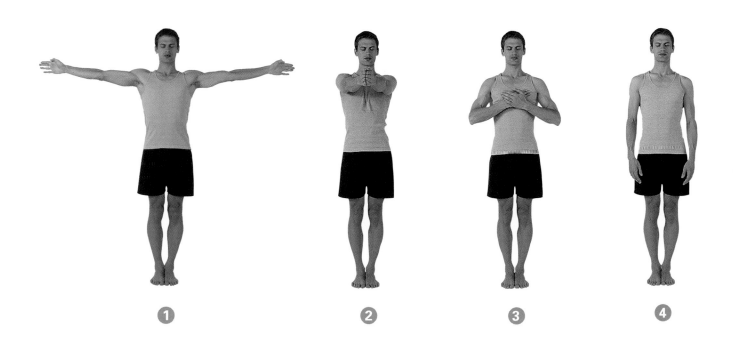

This kinesiology exercise simultaneously stimulates both hemispheres of the brain so that you think and move in a more coordinated way. It also helps to calm and balance the emotions by integrating confused and conflicting thoughts.

Try this in your lunch hour – ask your colleagues to join in too.

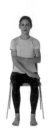

Yoga at work

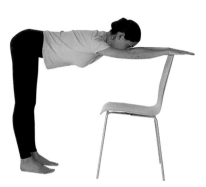
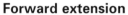

Forward extension

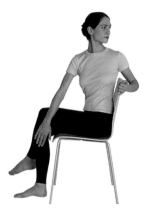

Spinal twist

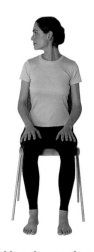

Head rotation

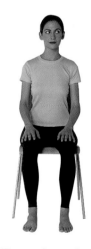

Eye relaxation

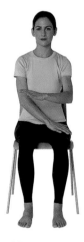

Knee taps

When you start to run out of energy at work or at home during the day, these simple yoga practices can be invaluable.

These postures are even more effective if you concentrate on your breath and allow your mind to clear.

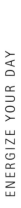

Forward extension Stand facing a chair. Bend and hold the back of the chair so that your legs are at 90 degrees to your body. Elongate your spine. Stretch your fingers.

Spinal twist Sit upright and cross your left leg over your right. Put your right hand over your left knee, your left hand on the chair back. Lift up your spine and twist your body to the left. Repeat on the other side.

Head rotation Sit or stand. Breathing out, turn your head to the right. Breathing in, return to center. Breathing out, turn to the left. Do this for 2 minutes.

Eye relaxation Imagine a clockface around your eyes. Look at 12 o'clock and count each numeral clockwise. Now do this counterclockwise. Repeat several times.

Knee taps Cross your arms and simply tap each knee in turn. Try to synchronize your breathing with the taps.

Vital sitting
at the end of the day

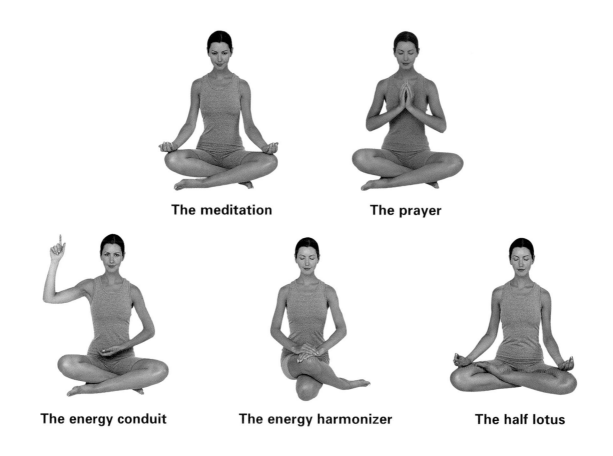

The meditation **The prayer**

The energy conduit **The energy harmonizer** **The half lotus**

The above qigong and yoga sitting postures open out the hip and shoulder girdles, increasing energy flow up the spine. Spend 5 minutes practicing one of them at the end of the day – close your eyes, breathe deeply and relax.

In sitting postures, when the hands are in an open position they receive energy; when they are held close to the body they conduct energy inward.

The meditation Sit cross-legged, keeping your spine straight (but not strained) and rest the backs of your hands on your knees.

The prayer Touch the tips of your fingers and the heels of your hands together in a prayer position to energize and nourish the heart chakra (*anahata*).

The energy conduit Point one index finger skyward to draw down *qi*, your wrist facing forward. Cup your other palm horizontally in front of your navel.

The energy harmonizer Sit on one heel with your upper leg crossed as far as possible over the lower leg, your hands on top of each other on your knee.

The half lotus Sit cross-legged and bring one foot up onto the opposite calf. Place your hands on your knees, keeping the palms open.

Evening practice

center yourself after the day

Here are some simple meditative practices. Take time in the evening to relax and let go of the day's events. Try to practice with "conscious awareness": observe your thoughts but do not allow them to take over. Instead of judging your performance, simply think: "Now I am practicing yoga." Start by sitting comfortably with your back straight.

Humming-bee practice Close your eyes and relax. Close the flaps of your ears with your index fingers. Imagine a humming bee inside your head. Breathe in. Breathe out and make the even, controlled noise of a humming bee. Repeat up to 5 times. This produces a meditational state and eases stress and insomnia.

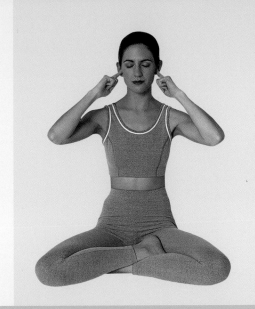

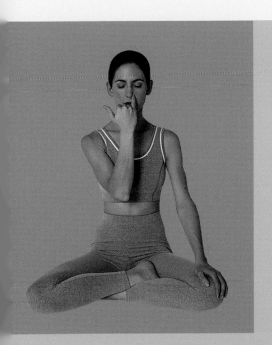

Alternate-nostril breathing Hold the right nostril closed with the thumb and breathe into the left nostril. Close the left nostril with the little finger, release the right nostril and breathe out. Breathe in through the right nostril, then close it with your thumb. Release your left nostril and breathe out. Repeat several times.

Visualization of chakras and colors Imagine drawing up red-colored energy from the earth into your base chakra. Visualize the color changes (red, orange, yellow, green, blue and violet) as the energy ascends the differently colored chakras. At the crown chakra the energy becomes white, creating an envelope around you.

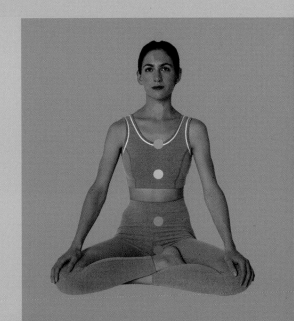

Bedtime relaxation

preparation for sleep

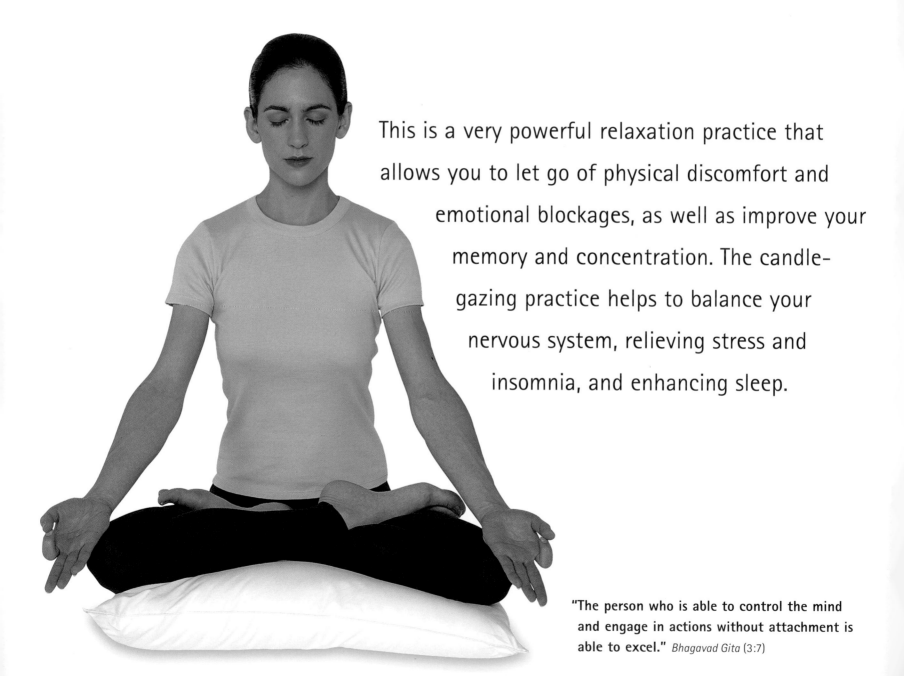

This is a very powerful relaxation practice that allows you to let go of physical discomfort and emotional blockages, as well as improve your memory and concentration. The candle-gazing practice helps to balance your nervous system, relieving stress and insomnia, and enhancing sleep.

"The person who is able to control the mind and engage in actions without attachment is able to excel." *Bhagavad Gita* (3:7)

Light a candle and your favorite incense. Spend a few minutes thinking over the events of the day and then let go of these thoughts. Make an agreement with yourself that for the next 15–20 minutes your thoughts will be on the practice of relaxation and meditation. Sit in a comfortable position with your back straight. Spend some minutes looking at the candle flame. Close your eyes and hold the image in your mind. When the image disappears, open your eyes and look at the flame again. Repeat this a few times.

Remain sitting or lie down on the floor in the relaxation pose, *shavasana* (see pp.48–49), but do not fall asleep. Practice yoga breathing (see pp.54–55) or alternate-nostril breathing (see p.123) for a few minutes and then scan your body, looking for tension. Breathe into any areas of tension and, when you breathe out, allow them to soften and release.

Now visualize the candle flame on the screen of your mind. Allow it to be small at first but, as you watch, see it grow bigger and brighter, washing over your body, bringing peace, love and compassion. Allow the flame to fill every aspect of your interior space and then let it focus at the heart chakra (*anahata*).

Allow this image to fade and bring your awareness to the breath at the tip of your nose. Then gradually become aware of your body, starting with your fingers and toes. When you are ready, gently open your eyes.

Sensing the energy

1 Stand, feet shoulders' width apart, knees slightly bent, arms by your sides. **2** Bring your hands in front of your abdomen, palms facing inward. Spend 2 minutes visualizing a ball of energy emanating from your abdomen, filling your hands. **3** Slowly, move your hands apart and imagine the ball of energy growing between them. Keep this position for 1 minute. **4** Now visualize the ball of energy contracting, as it pulls your hands in toward each other. Repeat several times until you can feel the energy expand and contract. **5** Draw your hands in toward your abdomen and imagine the ball of energy contracting back inside into a small spark. Wiggle your hands and shake your fingers.

ENERGIZE YOUR DAY

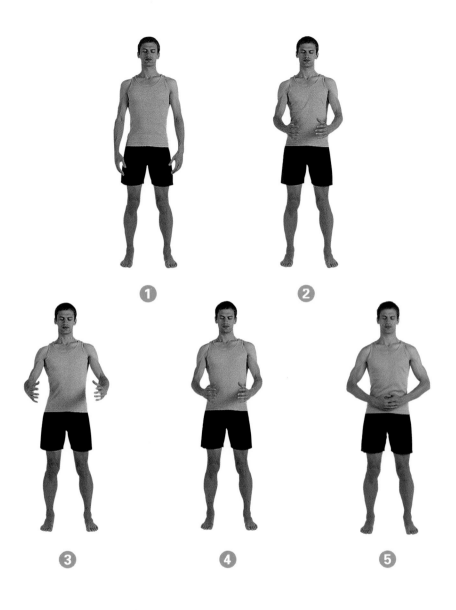

This qigong exercise can give you an energy boost at any time of the day. It helps to increase the flow in the energy center known as the lower dantien, which is located deep in the abdomen. According to Chinese tradition, the lower dantien is the seat of our being and the source of our vitality.

You will know when you succeed in feeling the energy between your hands – they will tingle or warm up.

Energy first-aid

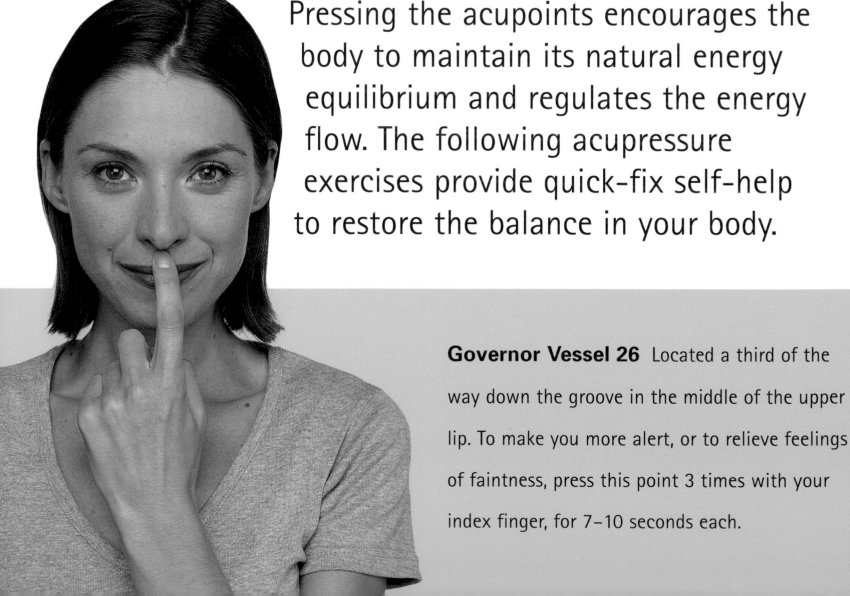

Pressing the acupoints encourages the body to maintain its natural energy equilibrium and regulates the energy flow. The following acupressure exercises provide quick-fix self-help to restore the balance in your body.

Governor Vessel 26 Located a third of the way down the groove in the middle of the upper lip. To make you more alert, or to relieve feelings of faintness, press this point 3 times with your index finger, for 7–10 seconds each.

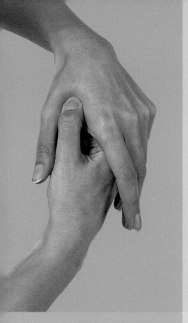

Large Intestine 4 Found in the fleshy web between the thumb and the index finger. Stimulating the energy flow in this meridian helps to treat diarrhea, rashes and toothache. Press this acupoint 3 times, on both hands, for 10–15 seconds each. It is not advisable to press this point on a pregnant woman.

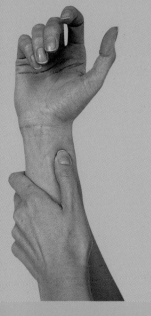

Lung 7 Located on the forearm, $1^1/_2$ in below the wrist fold, on the same side as the thumb, in the hollow behind the wrist bone. Pressing this acupoint helps to increase the energy flow to the lungs to combat respiratory problems, common colds and headaches. Press hard with your thumb 3 times, on both wrists, for 7–10 seconds each.

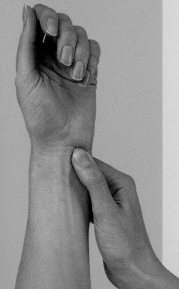

Heart 7 Found down below the little finger, on the inside of the wrist, just behind the wrist crease. Stimulating this acupoint helps to counteract irritability and to treat insomnia. Support your wrist with the fingers of your other hand, then press this point 3 times, on both wrists, for 7–10 seconds each.

Index

Acknowledgments

The Publishers would like to thank:

Models: Helen Brumby, Tim Cummins, Tara Fraser, Caroline Long, Kerry Norton

Make-up artists/hairdressers: Elizabeth Lawson, Evelynne Stoikou